Mudras

The Ultimate Guide to Mudras for Healing

(Simple Hand Gestures for Ultimate Memory Improvement)

Robert Wilson

Published By **Bella Frost**

Robert Wilson

Mudras: The Ultimate Guide to Mudras for Healing (Simple Hand Gestures for Ultimate Memory Improvement)

ISBN 978-1-998038-13-8

No part of this guidebook shall be reproduced in any form without permission in writing from the publisher except in the case of brief quotations embodied in critical articles or reviews.

Legal & Disclaimer

The information contained in this book is not designed to replace or take the place of any form of medicine or professional medical advice. The information in this book has been provided for educational & entertainment purposes only.

The information contained in this book has been compiled from sources deemed reliable, and it is accurate to the best of the Author's knowledge; however, the Author cannot guarantee its accuracy and validity and cannot be held liable for any errors or omissions. Changes are periodically made to this book. You must consult your doctor or get professional medical advice before using any of the suggested remedies, techniques, or information in this book.

Table Of Contents

Chapter 1: Meditation And Energy Healing Practices

Define Meditation & A Technique

The Process of Meditation is the exercising of turning your interest to a single point of reference. It can encompass focusing at the breath, on bodily sensations, or on a word or word referred to as a mantra. In different phrases, meditation manner the u . S . Of ZERO of the mind. The practices to obtain the dominion of Meditation is various but, the handiest is to have a take a look at your breath.

Main Physical Benefits of Meditation:

Decreases the bodily tension

 Delete psychosomatic issues due to anxiety

 Prophylaxis in competition to strain

 Lowers blood stress

 Strengthens the immune device

 It slows the developing older approach

1

Recharge our batteries

Main Psychological Benefits of Meditation:

Calm

Soothes, comforts

it permits to be more tolerant and sensitive

It allows to control our anger

Energizes

Take away the problems

Brings readability

It permits to be greater assured in ourselves

It lets in non-public increase

Some easy guidelines to start Meditating

– It is typically endorsed to try to meditate every day, probably on the identical time if you want to create a cutting-edge addiction.

– Do no longer meditate after food and pick out a time of day when you are not complete of electricity.

– Prepare the place in which you want to meditate, open a window to trade the air waft and if you need you can use a few incense.

– Choose a place no longer very vibrant, and put on cushty garments.

– It may be very vital that you are not disturbed during your meditation so disconnect your telephone, near the door and if that is the case, positioned a sign to in a polite manner ask not to be disturbed. It is a time of day committed to your self.

Technique:

Breath Meditation: Sit with out troubles in a posture. Clasp your hands and loosen up your every a part of your body. Now, supply all of your attention for your indoors and out breath. Anapanasati. Ana approach in, apana manner out and Sati technique turning into one with. Focus on your outside and inside breath and permit there be no distinctive interferences. Be with similar to hundreds as you can.

Elemental Meditation: Choose any detail from 5 (Air, Earth, Water, Fire & Space). Surround your self with the element of your desire and genuinely be there. Watch your feelings, thoughts and physical sensations. Be there with the enjoy as plenty as you can.

Body Meditation: Choose to be collectively with your frame and be there with it. Feel the presence of your frame at each element. Begin to transport beyond the layers of pores and skin. (Example: blood, organs, flesh, bones and so forth). Be with the go along with the flow as long as you may.

Environmental Meditation: Choose an area of your choice, in which you experience snug. Choose a posture and be there searching on the environment. Explore the region the manner you pick out to and the happenings if any. Observe the reactions of the frame at every level. Explore as deep as you may.

Sound Meditation: Choose a valid of your preference at the place you choice to art work. (Example: horror, Divine, Elements, Laughter, Pain and lots of others). Listen to the sound and witness the reactions of the frame. Feel the sensations at your heart. Be with this till it adjustments into special and the opportunity moreover modifications till you reach stillness.

Stillness Meditation: This is to stop your self wherein ever you are for your experience. Choose to be on the identical issue of cognizance. No adventure quarter. No idea and no feeling.

Tools of Inner Cleansing

Inner cleansing is the procedure of cleaning the pollution inside.

Deha and manas Shuddhi with Water.

Technique: Practical's with ingesting water (Naadi Shuddhi)

THIS IS THE EXERCISE THAT YOU WILL DO EVERYDAY FOR 10 MINS TO KEEP YOURSELF CLEANSED ALWAYS

Sit calm, snug, spine straight away, ideally in a chair. Keep the glass of water for your arms; be along side your ordinary breath. Focus to your breath until you are capable of be privy to the sound of the inhalation and exhalation. This is the issue one is prepared.

The relaxation of your aware worldwide has no employer this second, regardless of whom, what and why.

What you interest on, you energize it. Connect your self with the water. Keep the water glass very close to the nostrils and experience your breath inside the water. Thank the water; supply all of your gratitude.

The water cleanses, your inner, outer and your feelings proper from while you were born. Your mind may be acquired through way of the water. Release reason of cleaning all of the fears, guilt, beyond reminiscences, a few detail is applicable to you for my part. IF U HAVE PHYSICAL PAINS, contamination or any persistent disease, permit the cleaning energy cleanse your naadis or the pathway via which it'll tour from the whole intelligence keeping at once to the illness.

If you're searching out intellectual and emotional states of peace, love and happiness, there's an image of that within you. Sense the photo within the water and the tattwa shall deliver it via the naadis, or your existence pressure power or the praanic strength pathways to fill you with that that you are. You may even form your self bodily and mentally, via projecting the image of your healthful self into the water.

Whether it is diabetes, fever, cancer, depression, obesity or really cleansing for balanced emotional states or religious evolution, endure in thoughts that your motive might be passing via the pathways developing a beautiful template first of all and improvement closer to "that" with each excessive moment indoors.

So, permit's surely start

Your water is charged, at the side of your motive and readability and picture of in that you choice to reap. Take a sip of water, do now not gulp, and consciously consciousness on the possibly course. The water will excursion for your stomach, disconnect with some element else and slowly gulp the water sensing the nippiness of the water as it is going into your stomach. Now take a sip, close to your eyes, interest all your hobby to each of your ears and while no longer whatever else you're aware of, gulp the water sensing the relax of the water touching it or passing into it. Next, attention all your hobby to your eyes, take a sip, and as you gulp the water, revel in the coolness of the water soothing the eyes. Notice you're in reality sensing the tattwa of water in form of coolness and not imagining a few element.

Now attention all your hobby to the top of the top, and whilst you are absolutely there, take a sip and gulp the water sensing its movement on the top of the top. Next sip, enjoy the water power, or tattwa, or your reason passing thru from the lower back of the pinnacle, slowly down the spinal twine to the bottom of the Spinal Cord. Now you already got a sense of what you are doing.

Next step, consciousness all your attention to the entire decrease again and enjoy the chilliness of water soothing and a laugh as you enjoy its movement. You are pretty aware, that the water you take in is going on your stomach and now not to the areas which you are sensing. Yet it's far actual that you are sensing the motion of water during your frame. You have already consciously separated the hassle and power, at the identical time because the problem is going into the stomach; you're consciously able to revel in and ship energy wherein ever you need to through concept, consciousness and intent.

Now interest all of your interest onto your thighs. Be completely there. Take a sip, and gulp the water with complete interest at the thighs. You will experience the frenzy of power thru it. Focus next on the knees; Deeply, be there, take a sip, maintain on, gulp while you're truly there, you will experience the water tattwa passing thru the knees, soothing it. Shift all of your attention now to the bottom of the ft. Yes, experience the gravity, Sense the relationship. Take a big sip, slowly as you gulp the water experience the entire motion proper from the top of the top, down the spine, down the thighs, thru any effected region, into the bottom of the toes. The next sip, push the strength from the bottom of the ft into the earth, permit go all of the pain, the recollections. Just be there, breathing well and deep and experiencing the exhalation from the bottom of the ft into the earth.

You are completed.

You are aware that the water had clearly travelled into your stomach only, but it's miles your very very personal physical experience of the energies journeying a few course cleaning you, healing you.

One, who does naadishuddhi every day, shall revitalize the frame's natural functionality to heal itself, as it is cleansing itself regularly of all of the pointless sediments and keeps the breath smooth to get keep of from nature your due.

Mind Pollution: Technique:

Thoughts are your reminders of your reality. Look into all of the mind jogging prominently in you. Observe them. Are they brilliant or poor?

Useful or Useless? Choose one of the thoughts and begin to contemplate on it till it takes you to the subsequent degree and if it doesn't drop it for the time and choose out the subsequent distinguished one.

Open eye Process: Write down the maximum vital thoughts effective further to horrible. Prioritize and pick out the primary one and test out the significance of running with it now or later. If now, then start to ponder until it loses or improves its strength.

Practices of chakras, Naadis..

A chakra is a vortex of psychic power which may be visualized as circular movements of strength at a selected price of vibration. Physiologically, chakras are like junctions wherein the nerves meet and they may be located at the interior walls of the spinal column. They are like poles of energy, via which electric wires run for the duration of to supply energy at definitely one among a type facilities. Through the nerves praana or vital energy flows in advance and backwards.

The first of the chakras is referred to as the mooladhara (Root Center), it's located on the pelvic floor and it corresponds to the coccygeal plexus of the nerves. It is at this chakra that the focus rises above Animal Nature. Below this chakra there are imagined to be lower centers of power taking area to the heels, answerable for the growing the animal and the human traits of intuition and intellect. The mooladhara chakra controls the excretory and the sexual abilities inside the frame.

The 2d chakra called swadisthan lies on the terminal element of the spinal column. It relates to the sacral plexus of nerves and appears after the unconscious inside the character.

The Third chakra known as Manipura, lies at the backbone virtually on the Navel degree. It is related to the sun plexus and takes care of the digestive assimilative and the temperature manipulate systems of the frame.

The fourth chakra known as Anahata, is located within the vertebral column at the back of the coronary coronary heart close to the bottom and it is at the extent of the depression in the sternum. It is to the cardiac plexus of the nerves and takes care of the organ of the frame on this location which includes the coronary heart, the lungs, the diaphragm and so on.

The fifth center, called the Vishuddhi is situated in the vertebral column on the extent of the throat pit. It is related to the cervical plexus of the nerves and looks after the thyroid complex, top palate, epiglottis and many others.

The sixth chakra known as ajna is related to the pineal gland and is placed above the spinal column in the midline of the mind. It is the middle of command and appears after all of the capabilities of one's existence. In particular, it controls the sexual interest in the character.

The seventh chakras ia called the Sahasrara. It lies on the pinnacle of the pinnacle and is associated with the pituitary gland which is meant to take care of all the glands and systems of the body. Sahasrara is the seat of cosmic consciousness and is the terminal element of the adventure of Kunadalini shakti.

Mudras and Its Importance

The essence of mudras is to recognize that mudras supply route to the praana vayu.

What wants to be placed is the sound of the breath and the pressure of the breath as to

Where it's far wearing out. There in which till it reaches is the issue which it clears, energises and strengthens.

1. Observe breath with every fingers up - Observation have to experience one's presence in big element on the better a part of the frame.

2. Observe breath with each hands down – Observations need to experience one's presence on the lower a part of the body

3. Left palm up proper down - To the left aspect of the body

four. Left palm down, proper palm up (A few instances to clean sense the shift happenning) - To the right factor of the body

five. The thumb + Index finger - Largely at the pineal and pituitary glands ... Excellent for migraine patients.

This mudra is also called "Gyana Mudra" used in the path of meditations and rituals. This mudra helps to attain the levels of superconscious internal a quick term. It permits in developing information, reminiscence and awareness. The nerves of the mind get more potent and mind becomes calm and blissful.

6. The thumb+ index finger plus the middle finger - Thoracic gland... Exceptional for thyroid problem.

7. Thumb+ Middle finger pleasant- To anahata the heart chakra... Hypertension/ B.P Issues

eight. Thumb +Middle finger+ Ring finger- Manipuraka, indigestion, acidity, gasoline, uneasiness due to over consuming.

9. Thumb + ring finger handiest –Swadhisthan... Sensual problems, reproduction issues, emotional imbalance.

10 Thumb + Little finger - Mooladhara - releases fear, constipation, piles.

YOGA AND ITS TYPES

Define Yoga:

A Hindu religious and ascetic region, part of which, which include breath manage, easy meditation, and the adoption of specific physical postures, is broadly practiced for health and rest.

Yoga: Is Union. Union of energy and its rely. The entire advent is this. Eg: our meals. It's in united states of Yoga, a union of strength and its depend. Wherever there can be a union there can be additionally a separation. So, digestion is the technique that does this separation. The matter wide variety is going returned to wherein it came from and the electricity is utilized by the body. This have a have a look at of union and separation of energy and depend is the take a look at of Yoga.

Types of Yoga:

Hatha Yoga: Asana—posture: The zero.33 level at the eightfold path is referred to as Asana, which means that that, sincerely, posture. Some writers have tried to make the component that Patanjali refers proper proper right here to the want for schooling the yoga postures as a steerage for meditation. But Patanjali have become talking, no longer of practices, but of the outstanding tiers of non secular development. Here, then, posture way no particular set of postures, however simplest the potential to maintain the body however as a prerequisite for deep meditation. Any snug posture will do, as long as the spine is saved erect and the body snug. A signal of perfection in Asana is stated to be the capacity to take a seat down nonetheless, without moving a muscle, for 3 hours. Many human beings meditate for years without accomplishing any tremendous effects, genuinely because of the reality they have got by no means professional their our bodies to sit down however. Until the body may be mastered, better perceptions, so subtle that they blossom first-class in perfect quiet, can in no manner be completed.

It is good, of direction, to exercising some of the yoga postures in advance than meditation. These postures assist one to benefit Asana, or enterprise enterprise posture. Many starting college university college students, however, make the error of assuming that they must notable their exercise of the yoga postures in advance than even seeking to meditate. This is pretty unfaithful. It isn't always even essential to exercising the postures in any respect that allows you to observe meditation. The postures are fine an useful resource, even though a very tremendous one, to meditation

Mantra Yoga:

Mantra yoga is a kind of yoga that makes use of mantras to rouse the Self and deepen the meditative aspects of a bodily yoga exercise. Mantra yoga is an proper generation that is meant to engage the thoughts through that specialize in sound, duration and extensive fashion of repetitions. Repetition of the mantras is a method to get in the path of the divinity internal, and it creates extraordinary vibrations that advantage each the most effective who chants and the one who listens.

Mantra yoga can also be referred to as Japa yoga. Japa is a Sanskrit word for the act of repeating mantras. Mantra yoga neutralizes rajas (agitation) and tamas (inertia), which allows the practitioner to move right into a purer state of recognition. Chanting mantras calms the thoughts, brings interest and is exceptional for controlling the breath. Mantra yoga is especially useful to the practitioner because it improves traditional health and intellectual balance.

Although Mantra yoga is typically considered an innovation of Hinduism, it's been adopted and advanced via wonderful religions as properly. Religions like Buddhism and Jainism have embraced Mantra yoga as a part of their own efforts to reap enlightenment.

Mantra yoga may be practiced in 3 methods. The first manner is known as baikhari, in which the mantra is chanted in a loud manner. This shape of chanting is superb for disposing of undesirable thoughts from the thoughts with the intention to make the meditation method less difficult. The second method of chanting is referred to as upanshu, in which the mantra is chanted in a completely low voice that only the practitioner will pay interest. The zero.33 method is chanting the chant silently to one's self. This is known as manasic and it is utilized by advanced practitioners. Individuals can also like to use mala (yoga beads) to preserve rely of their repetitions.

Yantra Yoga:

Yantra Yoga is one of the oldest recorded systems of yoga in the international. It has come to us with the resource of way of Tibet, a land that holds a sizeable, wealthy Buddhist facts and facts. Yantra Yoga's precise series of positions and actions, mixed with conscious respiration, can assist coordinate and harmonize one's non-public electricity definitely so the mind can loosen up and find out its true balance. Many positions utilized in Yantra Yoga are just like those of Hatha Yoga, but the way to expect and take a look at them differs significantly. Yantra Yoga uses a sequence that consists of seven tiers of movement, related with seven ranges of respiratory. In precise, the area inside the critical segment of each motion enables create specific retentions of the breath that artwork at a deep, diffused level. For this reason, it isn't always simplest the precept position, but this maintaining and the whole movement which is probably crucial.

The machine of Yantra Yoga carries a large sort of actions that may be completed through everybody. It is a first rate approach for carrying out principal fitness, rest, and stability via the coordination of breath and motion. Although a Yantra Yoga practitioner does not usually want to observe a specific religious course, therefore everybody can workout it with out quandary

Bhakthi Yoga:

Bhakti yoga, additionally referred to as Bhakti marga (surely the direction of Bhakti), is a spiritual route or spiritual exercise internal Hinduism focused on loving devotion inside the path of a private god... It is one of the paths within the religious practices of Hindus, others being Jnana yoga and Karma yoga..

Tantra Yoga:

The phrase "tantra" literally manner a way or a generation. This is an inner technology. These are subjective techniques now not goal techniques. But within the modern-day knowledge in society, the phrase "tantra" refers to very unorthodox or socially unacceptable techniques. It is honestly that satisfactory factors are applied in a nice manner. It isn't always any distinct from yoga. It is a limb of yoga called tantra yoga.

The human mechanism is a composite of the physical body – an accumulation of meals fed on; the mental frame – the software program program application and memory issue that makes humans feature in unique techniques; and the power frame – the vital upon which the ones are housed. What is past that is non-bodily.

The compulsive and cyclical nature of the body and thoughts render themselves a barrier for better possibilities. Tantra is to transport past, without a doubt so compulsiveness of the frame and mind does now not maintain us trapped in our boundaries. It is about learning to apply the frame, not as oneself, but as a stepping-stone to supply this being to the very best possible size.

Tantra is not about unbridled sexuality, as assumed by means of using manner of many. Sexuality is a fundamental intuition instilled in our our our bodies to make certain the species perpetuates itself. This is a essential requirement. At the same time, one want to recognize the boundaries beyond which it'll no longer deliver us. It is best on spotting the restrictions and the longing to touch different dimensions enters, that yoga and tantra become relevant.

Tantra approach you are able to use your energies to make subjects take area. If you could make your mind razor sharp to reduce through the whole thing, that is additionally one shape of tantra. If you're making your energies art work upon your coronary heart to become absolutely loving and you could burst forth with considerable love that truely overwhelms all and sundry, this is additionally tantra. If you are making your bodily body as an alternative effective to make it do super feats, this is moreover tantra. Or if you could make your energies do topics via itself without the usage of the frame, mind or emotion, that is additionally tantra.

So tantra isn't a few weird nonsense. It is a first-rate capability. Without it there's no possibility. If all you want is to do a meditation or religious exercise, you don't really need a Guru. The Guru is here basically to overwhelm you with anonymous ecstasies. So tantra is a technology of liberation, now not enslavement.

Tan is the frame and tra method liberation. Liberating an expression from the body-mind-being complicated

may be understood as Tantra.

Karma Yoga:

Karma technique movement. An movement is like projection and each projection has a mirrored photo.... This game of Projection and mirrored image instigated with the useful resource of movement is called Karma... Karma becomes Yoga at the same time as Dharma or right purpose is its doer... The region of selfless motion as a way to perfection...

Your art work is your duty, no longer its give up end result... Never allow the quit end result of your movements,

be your motive. Nor supply in to us of a of no interest. Set firmly in yourself, do your artwork, now not related to whatever. Remain even minded in success, and in failure. Even mindedness is proper yoga. (Bagavad gita)

Dhyana—meditation or absorption

Dhyana Yoga:

The 7th diploma is called Dhyana, meditation, absorption. By extended recognition on any degree of recognition, one starts offevolved offevolved to count on to himself its features. By meditating on sense pleasures, the Inner Self entails pick out out its happiness with the gratification of these pleasures; the individual loses sight of the indwelling Self because the actual deliver of his pleasures. (If a few detail, cloth changed into without a doubt a purpose of happiness, it would purpose happiness to all guys. The fact that it does no longer proves that it is our reactions to those topics, in vicinity of the topics themselves, that supply us our enjoyment.) Again, thru interest on our non-public faults, we incredible provide strength to those faults. (It is a intense mistake constantly to call oneself a sinner, as many orthodox religionists might have one do. One need to supply interest to one-of-a-kind function if he could probable come to be virtuous.) By concentrating on the inner moderate, then, or upon every other divine fact that one in reality perceives at the same time as the mind is calm, one often takes at the traits of that inner reality. The thoughts loses its ego identification, and starts offevolved to merge inside the notable ocean of cognizance of which it is a part.

Dhyana method contemplation or focusing. Dhyana will become Yoga whilst one loses the difference the numerous item of meditation and the witness itself.

Gnana Yoga:

Gnana manner know-how. Knowledge outcomes in information and higher belief of what's. When Gnana or know-how turns into one's conviction it's miles Yoga attained with the information...

Ashtanga or "Eight-limbed" Yoga

Patanjali, the notable historical exponent of Raja Yoga, wrote that the direction to enlightenment embraces 8 degrees. (His training is also called Ashtanga, or "Eight-limbed," Yoga.) An rationalization of those 8 "limbs" will assist to provide an knowledge of the deeper functions and guidelines of yoga.

Yama and Niyama

The first tiers of Patanjali's eightfold course are known as Yama and Niyama. Yama manner manage; Niyama, non-manipulate. Literally, those stages imply the don'ts and the dos on the spiritual path. They are, one may additionally moreover say, the Ten Commandments of yoga.

Their essential purpose is to permit the milk of internal peace to be amassed inside the pail of the thoughts thru plugging holes which have been due to restlessness, wrong attachments, goals, and numerous types of inharmonious dwelling.

The hints of Yama (the Don'ts) are five:

Non-violence or Ahimsa

Non-mendacity

Non-stealing

Non-sensuality or Brahmacharya

Non-greed or Non-attachment

It is interesting to note that each one of those virtues are listed in terrible phrases. The implication is that after we put off our delusions, we can not but be benevolent, sincere, respectful of others' belongings, and plenty of others., because of the fact it's far our nature to be accurate. We act otherwise now not due to the fact it's far herbal for us to achieve this, however because of the reality we have got embraced an unnatural america of egoistical in harmony.

The policies of Niyama (the Do's) are:

Cleanliness

Contentment

Austerity

Self-examine or Introspection

Devotion to the Supreme Lord.

Pranayama—strength control

The fourth level of Patanjali's path is Pranayama ... Prana does suggest breathe, but simplest because of the close connection that exists most of the breath and the causative waft of strength inside the body. The word, prana, refers more often than not to the power itself. Pranayama, then, approach electricity control. This energy manipulate is frequently affected with the useful useful aid of respiratory wearing events. Hence, respiration sports activities have moreover grow to be known as pranayamas.

Patanjali's reference is to the electricity manipulate that is accomplished due to numerous strategies, and now not to the techniques themselves. His phrase indicates a country in which the electricity in the body is harmonized to the point wherein its go with the flow is reversed—no longer outward towards the senses, but inward in the direction of the Divine Self that lies inside the hearts of all beings. Only whilst all the strength inside the body can be directed in the direction of this Self can one's recognition be excessive sufficient to penetrate the veils of myth and enter extraordinary-attention.

The very strength with which we count on is the identical energy that we use to digest our food. To check this declare, recollect how tough it is, after a heavy meal, to reflect onconsideration on weighty troubles, and the way easy the thoughts becomes after a brief. To divert all the power from the body to the mind can't but accentuate one's focus, and the ardour of one is conscious. To direct this strength inwardly is the first step in divine contemplation.

Pratyahara—the interiorization of the thoughts

The 5th degree on Patanjali's adventure is known as Pratyahara, the interiorization of the thoughts. Once the strength has been redirected in the direction of its supply in the mind, one want to then interiorize one's interest, in order that his thoughts, too, will not wander in limitless bypaths of restlessness and myth, however may be targeted one-pointedly at the deeper mysteries of the indwelling soul. A thread must be accumulated to at least one point in advance than it is able to be put through the eye of a needle. Similarly with the mind: It is vital to pay attention one's thoughts in addition to one's energies, if he may also need to desire to penetrate the slender tunnel that results in divine awakening.

Dharana—contemplation

Patanjali's 6th degree is known as Dharana, contemplation, or steady inner recognition. One might also additionally had been aware about internal religious realities—the inner mild, as an example, or the inner sound, or deep mystical feelings—earlier than reaching this degree, but it's far quality after attaining it that one have to supply himself honestly to deep recognition on the ones realities.

Samadhi—oneness

The 8th step on Patanjali's eightfold journey is called Samadhi, oneness. Samadhi comes after one learns to dissolve his ego focus inside the calm internal moderate. Once the grip of ego has absolutely been damaged, and one discovers that he's that moderate, there may be now not anything to prevent him from increasing his attention to infinity. The devotee in deep Samadhi realizes the truth of Christ's terms, "I and my Father are one." The little wave of slight, dropping its delusion of separate existence from the sea of slight, becomes itself the big ocean.

Siddhis

These are the powers which the practitioner receives relying at the spiritual growth. They are:

•Anima- The functionality to pay attention all the strength or prana inside the frame to at least one region that allows you to obtain the power of reducing the scale of the body to any degree. The goddess of this siddhi is Indrani.

Mantra- Om Aim Indraaniyai Namo Namaha (108 repetitions)

Chapter 2: Meditation And Its Stages

Mind to no thoughts

Consciousness – Witnessing – Awareness

Consciousness = "Sense of Presence" = "The Beingness" = The "I AM"

Witnessing is a courting amongst problem and item. Witnessing is a state; cognizance is a way inside the path of witnessing. The herbal attention is in truth the, without which there may be no attention.

Savitarka/ Gross

 Savichara/ Certain

 Sananda/ Bliss

 Sasmita/ I-ness

 Asamprajnata/ Objectless

Ana-pana-sati/ Vipassana

Ana-pana-sati

Ana = inhalation, Pana = Exhalation, Sati = merging into one

Kayanuppassana technique Complete focus on Body. Focussing on each a part of the body and its moves.

Vedananupassana method statistics the emotions and its nature of intensity.

Chittanupassana way beings with recognition. At a degree in which one will become a being with interest. Focussing on interest or being aware about the Self in all elements.

Dhammanupassana manner information thoughts. Knowing the perceptions, authenticity, integration and perspectives of thoughts working mechanism.

Vipassana method being insightful. Out give up give up end result of converted transformation.

Nirvana approach absolute. Objectless.

Recapitulations

The Science of Meditation

What is Meditation?

Meditation is a "No-mind State"; Chitta Vritti Nirodha… It is genuinely going on… Emptying the thoughts from all the thoughts… Making mind like an empty bowl… Meditation is witnessing the sports of self or cognizance… It is letting waft and a everyday workout of mindfulness of breath… It is non-doing and is living inside the now and proper right here being simply silent and nonetheless, awakening oneself to altered states of recognition… Meditation is silencing the inner speak and making contact with our internal essence…

What isn't always Meditation?

Meditation isn't always an intellectual system, nor a intellectual exertion… It isn't always popularity, prayer, worship or contemplation… Neither meditation is chanting of mantras or any visualization… Meditation isn't thoughts control…

Myths and Misconceptions about Meditation

Meditation is simplest for vintage human beings and one wishes to visit woodland or mountains for meditation… One desires a supervision of a

Guru for meditation and it is an break out from worldly responsibilities... It is hard to meditate... Meditation is best for religious humans and it requires renunciation and is a intense affair... Meditation detaches from dreams and feelings and is all approximately relaxation...

How to Meditate?

Get into a cushty posture

Clasp your hands

Cross your legs (if sitting in a chair)

Close your eyes

Observe the natural float of your breath...

When to Meditate?

Meditating on the same time each day is awesome

However, on every occasion is terrific...

Where to Meditate?

Any location is the proper place

Meditating inside the equal location each day is first-rate

How extended to Meditate?

Minutes of 1's age… (25 minutes, if 25 the age)

Meditational Experiences

Physical Experiences – Pain in the body elements, Itching, Head falling beforehand and backward, Bodily jerks, contractions and spasms, Body tremors, Body Swaying, Physical restlessness, Body turning into heavy and Light, Immobility, Physical Warmth, Sweating, Cold Shivers, Trembling, Goosebumps, Sensation of falling, Yawning, involuntary sighing, coughing, spontaneous alignment of backbone, upward rolling of eye balls, numbness, mystical sounds of Om, bells, drums, veena, conch, flute and so on., Buzzing, hissing, thunder sounds, sounds of ocean waves and waterfalls, seeing tremendous lighting fixtures, seeing colorations, vision of deities, lightening of the sector of focus, divine fragrances, sweet taste in mouth, feeling of breeze on pores and skin, tingling sensation at the brow or crown of the pinnacle, spontaneous rapid respiration, spontaneous stopping of breath, growth of frame, losing focus of frame from neck downwards, levitation…

Mental Experiences – Mental restlessness, resistance, resenting the method, improved mind, reduced mind, taking component within the technique, no thoughts, dropping recognition of time, unconscious sleep…

Emotional memories – Feelings of pleasure, tears flowing, and emotions of peace…

Energy Experiences – Raised vibrations, feel of ecstasy and blissfulness, feeling of electricity moving internal backbone…

Astral Experiences – Spontaneous beyond lifestyles do not forget, seeing future sports happening within the now, tunnel stories, astral tour, communique with spirit publications and angels, sounds and photographs of various geographical areas, out of frame reviews, superior psychic visions…

Deep Spiritual Experiences – Connection with the supply, complete stillness/Samadhi,

Receiving excellent consciousness, concept and insights...

Seven our bodies/ Koshas

Annamaya Kosha/Physical – Occupies time and region, Food sheath – Right food

Pranamaya Kosha/Etheric – Travels via space, Prana Sheath – Conscious practices

Manomaya kosha/Astral – Travels through location and time (most effective person past), Mental Sheath – High top notch thoughts

Vigyanamaya kosha/Causal – Travels via place and time (beyond and future of the character), Knowledge Sheath – Right expertise

Anandamaya Kosha/Spiritual – Travels through time (past and future of everyone), Bliss Sheath – Living in pride

Vishwamaya Kosha/Cosmic – Cosmic oneness, Cosmic Sheath – Practicing Oneness

Nirvanamaya Kosha/Nirvanic – Nirvanic Sheath – Zero Point Field

Meditation & Third Eye Experiences

The moderate of the body is the eye; consequently, thy eye be unmarried, thy complete body can be whole of mild.

Once we begin to exercise meditation, we start getting unique styles of reviews… Most of those studies can be categorised as "Third Eye Experiences".

"Third Eye Experiences" are the studies of our inner senses/extra sensory belief/non-physical senses…

How does Meditation result in "Third Eye Experiences"?

The First Happening – When we're with the normal, herbal, simple, smooth, gentle, gentle, shallow, tranquil, non violent flow of breath, the thoughts becomes as an possibility empty…

The Second Happening – When the mind is instead empty, massive quantity of cosmic power enters the bodily body…

The Third Happening – When sufficient quantity of cosmic electricity enters the physical frame, the end result is an cheaper quantity of activation of the 1/three eye…

Thus, Meditation effects in activation of our "inner senses" or the "0.33 eye". The give up stop end result of meditation is activation of our more sensory perception…

Physical Sensations related to Third Eye Experiences

Tingling feelings at the brow

Sense of Pressure on the middle of the forehead

Pain in the forehead area

Itching and pulling sensation within the fore head place

Chapter 3: Meditation And Seven Energy Centers

Purusha And Prakruti

The concept of "Purusha" and "Prakruti" from ancient Vedic expertise is a captivating concept… According to which, the universe consists of 2 components; The Manifest and the Un-appear Universe… The Un-occur is the natural hobby it honestly is the essence of the universe and is referred as "Purusha". When interest intends to take location some thing and directs its interest toward it, it manifests… The limitless manifestations, that we see within the universe originate from the same attention and shape the take place universe and is called "Prakruti". "Purusha" is the seed or capability and "Prakruti" is the fruit or "Kinetic". Everything begins offevolved from the deliver and returns to supply, and no longer in advance than it has found out its endless functionality and its "oneness" with deliver… The tool of interest is what we time period as evolution… There exist electricity facilities interior us which might be related to deliver… The awakening and growth of these power centers lead us to our reunification with supply... Meditation turns

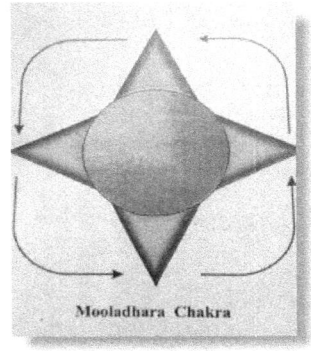

Mooladhara Chakra

on those centers...

The Six Chakras and the Seventh State

1.Mooladhaara Chakra – Physical identity, Focus-survival...

Located a number of the anus and the genitals and is established with the coccyx (a Triangular bone at the bottom of the backbone). Associated with Earth Element... It affords the inspiration for our existence in bodily truth... It is related to our survival instincts, and to our revel in of grounding and connection to our our our our bodies and the physical aircraft... When

43

activated, this chakra brings us fitness, prosperity, safety and dynamic presence…

About Mooladhaara Chakra:

- Main problem: Physical goals

- Form of Yoga: Hatha Yoga

- Sensory Function: Smell

- Element: Earth

- Mode of Sleep: On belly 10 to 12hrs

- Associated Glands: Adrenals

- Associated Body Parts: Spine, Bones, Teeth, Nails, Cell Multiplication, Skeletal System

- Location: Between anus and Genitals

- Archetypes: Elephant

- Physical Dysfunction: Osteoarthritis

- Emotional Dysfunction: Mental Lethargy

- Life Lesson: Standing up for oneself

- Goals: Physical fitness and Fitness, Stability and Security

•Fears: To Trust, Abandonment, Undeservability, Self-Destructive

•Traumas: Birth Trauma, Unconscious Death Urge

•Reflections: Reflection of Parent/Creator

•Character Structure: Schizoid

•Financially: Helplessness

•Sutra to be discovered: The Sutra of Abundance

•Positive Poles: Surrenderness, Sacrifice, Willingness

•Too Open: Overly Materialistic

•Blocked: Emotionally Needy

•Balanced: Emotional Mastery, Grounded, Healthy

Motto : Unconditional Acceptance

Technique :

Sit preferably in a dark room with eyes closed on a rug. Breathe normally for a few minutes feeling that each a part of the frame is getting comfortable. Continue to breathe normally, location the arms in "Gyana mudra" on the knees.

1.Inhale and exhale deeply for a rely of a hundred. With every inhalation and exhalation sense all the tensions flowing out and the body being energized from the inflow of the breath.

2.Relax for a minute.

3.Inhale deeply and pull the anus up closer to the bottom of the spine. The tongue need to the touch the palate.

four.Concentrate at the place of mooladhara.

5.Contract all of the muscle groups of the perineum and keep the breath for half a minute. Release and hold the breath. Repeat the method for four instances. This will help in know-how the feeling of mooladhar chakra.

6.During the relaxation of the device, respiration need to be deep.

7.See the 4 petal lotus rotating anti-clockwise route on the area of the chakra. The pace of rotation of this chakra will boom slowly. Feel the warmth spreading at some stage in the genital location.

8.Mentally chant the chant "Lam" inside the middle, "Vam" inside the proper, "Sham" going through downwards, "Sham" in the left and "Sam" dealing with upwards.

9.As you chant the ones mantras, experience the vibration and sensations going up from the lowest of the backbone to the crown.

10. When your breathing turns into heavy and deep, prevent and slow all of the manner all of the way all the way down to normal.

11. Contract all the muscle tissues of the perineum and hold the breath for 1/2 of a minute.+ Release the muscles and the breath. Repeat four instances.

12. Repeat the decision "Mooladhar Uthana" three times at the same time as focusing on the chakra.

2.Swadhishtana Chakra – Emotional identification, Focus-Desire...

It is positioned over the spleen and is related to the element water... Related to feelings and sexuality... It connects us to others via feeling, preference, sensation and movement... When activated, this chakra brings us fluidity and style, depth of feeling, sexual success and the capability to virtually get hold of exchange...

About Swadhisthaana Chakra:

•Main Issue: Emotional balance, Sexuality

•Form of Yoga: Bhakti Yoga

•Sensory Function: Taste

•Element: Water

•Mode of Sleep: Prenatal Position 8 to 10hrs

•Associated Glands: Ovaries, Testes,

Reproductive System

•Associated Body Parts: Sex Organs, Bladder,

Womb

•Location: Upper part of Sacrum, Upper restrict of Pubic Hair

- Archetype: Fish Tailed Alligator

- Physical Dysfunction: Impotence, Frigidity, Lower Back Pain

- Emotional Dysfunction: Unbalanced Sex Drive, Feelings of Isolation, Emotional Instability

- Life Lesson: Challenging Motivations based totally totally on Social Conditioning

Goals: Allowing Pleasure, Creative Expression

- Fears: Self-Deprecation, Not Worthy, Unlovability

- Traumas: Parental Disapproval Syndrome, Specific Negatives

- Reflections: Reflections of most Forgotten Love

- Character Structure: Masochist

- Relation with Money: Concern

- Sutra to be followed: The Sutra of Flow

- Positive Pole: Humility, Openness, Soft Spoken

- Too Open: A fantasist, Sexually Addictive

•Blocked : Frigid, Hard on Self, Feels Guilty

•Balanced: Trusting, Expressive, Tuned to Self-emotions, Creative

Motto: Attitude of Gratitude

Technique:

 The outstanding time to do this meditation is the night time time actually before the sundown. Sit dealing with the west route.

1.Start with the strength burst workout. This is also referred to as "Kapalabatti" and is an art work of respiratory practiced to purify the respiratory, circulatory and the digestive device.

2.Relax for a minute or .

three.Place the right hand above the pubic bone and left hand at the coronary coronary heart chakra. The pubic bone is the bodily vicinity of the swadhishthana chakra.

4.Inhale and exhale deeply.

5.Mentally repeat "Swadhishthana Uthana" three instances.

6.Now area every the arms to your knees in gyana mudra and close to your eyes.

7.Visualize six petal lotuses on the vicinity of the chakra. See the petals rotating in clockwise path. As the rotation profits tempo, sense the nippiness spreading in some unspecified time in the future of the pubic area.

8.Mentally chant the mantra "VAM" on the

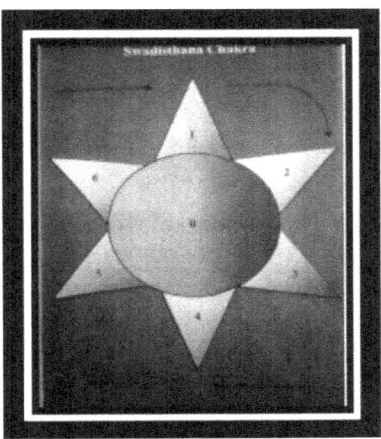

middle and "BAM", "BHAM", "MAM", "YAM", "RAM", "LAM", flowing from the elements 1 to

Chapter 4: About Manipura Chakra

•Physical Dysfunction: Stomach Ulcers, Diabetes, Allergies

•Emotional Dysfunction: Oversensitive to Criticism, Need to be on top of things, Low Self Esteem

•Main Issue: Personal energy, self Will

•Form of Yoga: Tantra Yoga

•Sensory Function: Sight

•Element: Fire

•Mode of Sleep: On again 7 to 8hrs

•Associated Glands: Pancreas

•Associated Parts of Body: Digestive System, Autonomic Nervous System

•Location: Two hands above the Navel

•Archetype: Spiritual Warrior

•Life Lesson: Self-Esteem/Self-Confidence, Courage to take dangers

•Goals: Purpose, Effectiveness, Self-Respect

- Fears: Arrogance, Loneliness, Greed

- Traumas: Senility, Past Life Trauma

- Reflections: Reflections of Judgment

- Character Structure: Psychopath

- Relation with Money: Hopelessness

- Sutra to be Followed: Sutra of Attention

- Positive Poles: Pride, Being Independent, Self-Assured, Abundant

- Too Open: Angry, Workaholic, Judgmental,

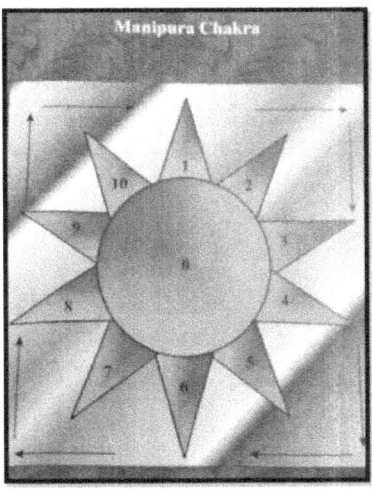

Superior

•Blocked: Overly Concerned with what others count on, Fearful of being on my own, Insecure

•Balanced: Respects self and others, Has personal electricity, Spontaneous

•Motto: Self Love

Chapter 5: Technique

This Saadhana is incredible finished in the afternoon, going thru the japanese side.. One can also do it outdoor at some point of wintry weather season..

Sit successfully in sidhaasana with arms in gyana mudra

Do nadi-shuddhi pranayam for five mins..

Relax for a fast whilst..

Place your right hand on the navel location and the left straight away within the lower lower back of the navel vicinity.. This is the vicinity for the manipura chakra..

Inhale deeply and exhale... Hold the breath for a few seconds...

Repeat the manner for ten minutes concentrating at the manipuraka chakra...

Mentally chant the mantra "om mani padme hum" seven times...

Place your hands once more on the knees in gyaana mudra or the mudra of the chakra...

Mentally see the chakra rotating in the clock realistic direction…

Feel the chakra rotating and gaining pace – the body receives hotter…

See the bheeja mantra "RAM" within the center of 10 petals…(others DAM DHAM NAM THAM THAM DHAM NAM PAM FAM)

Take a deep breath; Hold the breath for a minute, exhale… Repeat the method…

Mentally chant "Manipura Uthana" three instances…

Technique 2:

Sit in siddhaasana preferably with gyaana mudra..

Raise your head little upwards…

Inhale and exhale deeply… As you inhale say "am no longer the frame" and as you exhale say "Am now not even the thoughts"… Repeat this for 15 minutes…

Now utter the phrase "AAAAAAAA……" little loud for few times… (Till you sense the sensations inside the stomach location)

Allow the cosmic go with the drift and stay in silence as long as you may…

4.Anahata Chakra – Social Identity, Focus- Acceptance

Located inside the middle of the breasts on the extent of region (region round) of the coronary coronary heart hollow space and is related to the element air… This chakra is associated with love, and is the integrator of opposites inside the psyche: Mind and frame, Male and woman, man or woman and shadow, ego and group spirit… This chakra allows us to love deeply, enjoy compassion, have a deep experience of peace and centeredness…

About Anahata Chakra

•Main Issue: Beliefs approximately Love & Relationships

•Form of Yoga: Karma Yoga

•Sensory Function: Feeling

- Element: Air

- Mode of Sleep: On left aspect 5 to six hrs

- Associated Glands: Thymus

- Associated Parts of Body: Circulatory device, Heart and Chest, Lungs

- Location: Center of the chest

- Archetype: Antelope

- Physical Dysfunction: Shallow breathing, High B.P, Cancer, Heart illness

- Emotional Dysfunction: Fears about betrayal, Co-dependant, Melancholic

- Life Lesson: Forgiveness and Compassion

Goals: Balance, Compassion, Self-popularity

- Fears: Impatience

- Traumas: Past Karmas

- Reflections: Reflection of loss

- Character Structure: Rigid

- Relation with Money: Anger

•Sutra to be Followed: Sutra of Intention

•Positive Poles: Acceptance, Compassion, Selflessness

•Too Open: Possessiveness, Conditioned, Overly Dramatic

•Blocked: Fears Rejection, Loves an excessive amount of, Unworthy, Self-pity

•Balanced: Compassionate, Unconditional, Desires spiritual revel in in Love Making

Motto: Unconditional Love

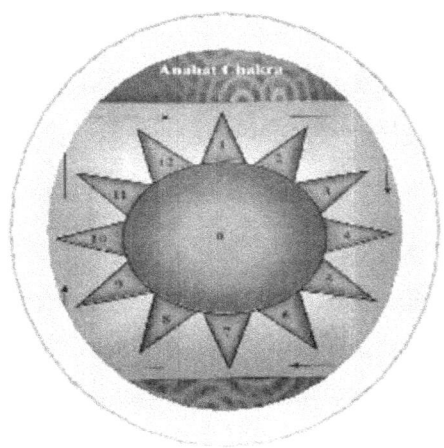

Technique

1.Sit effects in siddhasana with folded fingers on the coronary coronary coronary heart. Close your eyes and breathe typically.

2.Bring your popularity to the chest and enjoy the growth and contraction with each breath. Be on this attention for ten minutes.

three.Do the internal voice approach. Hands in Gyana mudra or mudra of the chakra.

four.Relax for a minute or two.

5.Do self introspection technique.

6.Place the proper hand at the chest and the left hand at the lower part of the chest.

7.Visualize the given diagram on the coronary heart location and enjoy the chakra rotating.

eight.Sense the beej mantra "YAM" in the center of the chakra. Feel it with emitting golden mild that fills you up with divine emotions. The exceptional petals of the chakra have the subsequent mantras: KAM, KHAM, GAM, GHAM, DAM, CHAM, CHAM, JAM, JHAM, TRAM, TAM, and THAM.

9.Mentally chant "Anahata Jagrate" seven instances bringing the notice to the coronary heart.

10. Do the self introspection all over again. Relax.

eleven. Repeat "Anahat Uthana" 3 instances.

This meditation is accomplished for each week or more to awaken the Anahata. After the awakening, a person turns into humble, noble, and knowledgeable and gets a radiance of spirituality.

Self Introspection:

Close your eyes and breathe normally for a few minutes till you get a sense of the go with the flow of the breath inner. Let the inhalation float through your frame and touch every a part of the body. You're respiratory pattern and its commentary lets in to obtain the deeper ranges of meditation. When you breathe normally, be aware that the breath goes in proper till the stomach at each inhalation and out from the stomach via the nostril at each exhalation.

This workout will heighten your inner capabilities to transport on within the pathless route. Do this in absolute silence.

Inner Voice Technique

Sit in siddhasana in gyana mudra. Close your eyes. With each breath you inhale and exhale, experience the energy flowing thru your device making you entire of white moderate. Release all the horrible thoughts as you breathe out.

Take a deep breath out of your nose and maintain the breath. Take your right hand up and location the top of the thumb within the proper ear, index and center finger on the eye, ring finger on right nostril and little finger at the proper side of the lips. Repeat this with the left hand taking identical steps.

When all the senses are blocked, you may pay attention now not some thing inside the starting but will slowly begin listening to the sounds in the frame. Chant "OM" mentally till you are doing this. You may additionally begin with little time and increase step by step the duration. This workout will assist you advantage stability over your mind by using way of shutting all of the external distractions.

five.Visuddhi Chakra – Creative Identity, Focus-Creativity

Located some of the despair inside the neck and the larynx, (the hollow muscular organ forming an air passage to the lungs and defensive the vocal cords in people and first-rate mammals; the voice field) starting at the cervical vertebrae (Seven Cylindrical Bones or vertebral our bodies.. The vertebral frame is the huge part of the bone that lies anterior (in the front of) the spinal twine) within the again of the Adam's apple (a projection at the the the front of the neck customary through the thyroid cartilage of the larynx, frequently brilliant in guys)... Associated with the detail Ether, this chakra is associated with creativity and expression... All advent and expression begins offevolved from empty place due to the fact the universe have become created out of no-thingness... Thought, phrase and deed are the ranges of creation... Word represents the expression of purpose, it truly is a completely vital step inside the modern approach...

VISHUDDHI CHAKRA

• Main Issue: Communication, Self-expression

• Form of Yoga: Mantra Yoga

• Sensory Function: Hearing

• Element: Ether

• Mode of Sleep: Alternatively right and left additives

• Associated Glands: Thyroid, Para thyroid

• Associated Parts of Body: Respiratory tool, Esophagus, Nape of neck, Jaws

• Location: Between inner collar bone and Larynx

• Archetype: Bull

• Physical Dysfunction: Sore Throat, Neck pain, Thyroid Problems, Tinnitus, Asthma

• Emotional Dysfunction: Perfectionism, Inability to specific feelings, Blocked Creativity

•Life Lesson: Power of preference, Personal expression

•Goals: Harmony with others, Self records, Creativity

•Fears: Stubbornness

•Traumas: Expression

•Reflections: Quest into darkness

•Character Structure: Rigid

•Relation with Money: Anxiety

•Sutra to be Followed: Sutra of Gratitude

•Positive Poles: Determination, Fixedness of Purpose

•Too Open: Over Talkative, Dogmatic, Self-Righteous, Arrogant

•Blocked: Holds once more from self expression, Unreliable, Holds Inconsistent Views

•Balanced: Good communicator, Contented, Finds clean to meditate, Artistically Inspired

•Motto: Creative Expression

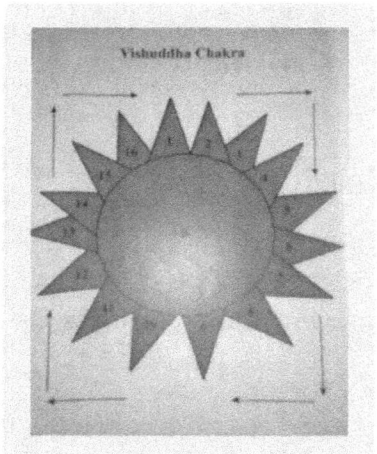

Technique

This Sadhana is best completed in advance than sundown. The following subjects used for this meditation:

•Spoonfull of Sandal powder

•Three spoons of rose water

•Few drops of aroma oil

•Two candles

•Make a wonderful paste via manner of blending the sandal powder, rose water and oil.

66

•Sit down in Siddhasana going through the north direction. The spine ought to be erect and arms in Gyana mudra.

•Do the internal invocation approach and lighten up for a minute.

•Use the proper hand first and the middle finger to attract the "Trishul" symbol inside the the front of you at the floor and place the 2 lighted candles inside the front of your knees. Place each the fingers at the photograph in such a way that the middle lining is also blanketed.

•Chant "Vishuddhi Jagratey" seven instances concentrating at the picture.

•Move your proper hand to the lump of the throat area even as letting the left hand be wherein it end up at the image.

•Massage the throat region with the proper hand transferring up and down. As you flow your right hand up and down, circulate your left hand inside the equal rhythm to the right and left on the image.

•Repeat the above gadget for a minute or so. This is the physical feature of the Vishuddhi and if the approach is achieved properly, you will enjoy the scent of sandal emitting from the throat chakra.

•Bring every the hands close to the lighted candles in one of these manner that the center of the fingers feels warm temperature. Chant "Vishuddhi Jagratey" seven instances, concentrating on the photograph.

•Close your eyes and see the chakra rotating. Chant "Vishuddhi Uthana" three times with beej mantra "HAM" inside the middle.

•The unique nadi mantras for this chakra are AM, AAM, IM, EEM, UM, UUM, REH, REEM, LRIM, LREEM, EIYM, EEYIM, OM, AUM, AM, AAH on the positions 1-sixteen respectively.

•Inhale deeply – keep the breath – chant 'Vishuddhi Uthana' another time for 3 times and forcefully enhale from the mouth to blow the candles off.

6.Ajna Chakra – Archetypal identification, Focus-seeing the massive photograph

Associated with the pineal gland, it truly is a completely small, shapeless organ, about 1/eight inch in diameter placed inside the forehead about one finger above the bridge of the nostril, among the two eyebrows… This chakra is not associated with any detail; it's far related to the capability of seeing the un-seem… It represents the potential to peer the entirety as part of a extra entire…

AJNA CHAKRA

•Main Issue: Intuition, Wisdom

•Form of Yoga: Jnana Yoga

•Sensory Function: All senses collectively with E.S.P

•Element: Light

•Mode of Sleep: Deep and 1/2 extensive extensive wakeful sleep For 4hrs

•Associated Glands: Pituitary

•Associated Parts of Body: Eyes, Base of Skull

•Location: Above & Between Eyebrows

- Archetype: None

- Physical Dysfunction: Headaches, Poor vision, Neurological Disturbances, Glaucoma

- Emotional Dysfunction: Nightmares, Learning problems, Hallucinations

- Life Lesson: Emotional Intelligence

- Goals: Ability to appearance apart from with the eyes

- Fears: Inner silence, Success

- Sutra to be Followed: Sutra of Gratitude

- Positive Poles: Determination, Fixedness of Purpose

- Too Open: Highly Logical, Dogmatic, Authoritarian, Arrogant

- Blocked: Undisciplined, Tendency within the path of schizophrenia, Sets elements of interest too low

- Balanced: Charismatic, Highly intuitive, Not connected to fabric topics, May revel in uncommon phenomenon

•Motto: Wisdom

Techinique-

TRATAK – THE WAY OF THE YOGI

This workout is fantastic executed within the night time time time or earlier than dawn. At a distance of two feet area a lighted candle on a desk on this sort of way that the slight og the candle is in right angles to the center of the eye

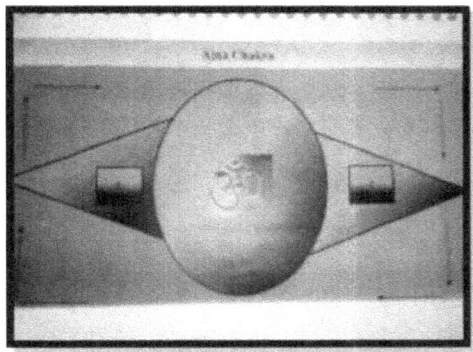

or the 'bhu madhya'.

STEP 1-

Tratak is a amazing 'thoughts controlling' tool and is utilized by all the yogis within the making.

The method of doing this 'kriya' is to first appearance on the tip of the flame for a minute with out blinking. When you experience you can't stare anymore, rub each your hands till you experience the warm temperature within the fingers- them vicinity your hands on the eyes and relax.

Again open the eyes and stare on the Candle. Close eyes with palms – take your eye balls to the 'bhu madhya' and visualize the candle flame burning here together with your inner vision revel in the warmth of the flame at the zero.33 eye. Open the eyes – see the candle- over again close to the eyes and visualize the flame inner.

Chapter 6: Calling To The Universal Soul

Do the internal invocation:

It is an exercising to invoke the energies the various coronary coronary coronary heart chakra and the Ajna Chakra.

Sit in Siddhasana with the once more straight, close to your eyes and take deep breaths. Each breath should be taken slowly with the feeling of the waft of the breath within the body.

a)With every breath you inhale experience the drift of the cosmic energy going in the body and lighting fixtures up all your frame structures.

b)Every breath you exhale feels the outflow of vain mind and tensions out of your frame.

c) Place your palms upwards in Gyana mudra preserving your lower back at once, decrease your head in this kind of manner that the chin touches the joint of the neck. Press the top within the course of the joint and skip on taking deep breathing following the identical sample as has been noted. This workout is right for invoking the power between the coronary

coronary coronary heart chakra and the ajna chakra.

After having practiced this for a while, go to a sophisticated degree in which you need to inhale deeply as has been accomplished in advance, and then, maintain the breath for a count number wide variety variety of and visualize that each one the strength is seeping into every part of the frame. Then exhale moreover within the identical way as has completed earlier.

Calling to the standard soul:

•Repeat A, B, C of the above.

•Keeping your lower back right away until your head closer to the lower back in a manner that the decrease again of the top touches the once more of the neck joint.

•Press the top in opposition to the joint and move on taking deep breath following the same sample as has been mentioned in A and B. This workout is right for the invocation of the energy among the Vishuddhi chakra and the Ajna Chakra.

•After having practiced this for a while, drift on the advanced stage and keep to the depend of two between inhalation and exhalation.

Precautions:

•Both the 1 and more than one carrying events involve the neck place so people struggling cervical spondalitis want to are seeking out advice from the health practitioner in advance than doing those.

•Never supply a jerk while transferring the top beforehand and backward.

Advantages:

•These physical activities close to the Ida and the Pingala nadis and inspire the glide of prana from the Shushumna nadi.

7.The sahasraara Chakra is known as the Crown Chakra – Universal Identity, Focus-Nirvana

It is absolutely a state of pure reputation… This country isn't associated with any element and pertains to recognition as natural attention… Represents the kingdom of consciousness of being one with all this is…

SAHASRAAR CHAKRA

- Main Issue: Spirituality

- Element: Thought, Cosmic power

- Mode of Sleep: Half Awake

- Associated Glands: Pineal

- Associated Parts of Body: Upper Skull,

Cerebral cortex, Skin

- Location: Top of the Head

- Archetype: None

- Physical Dysfunction: Sensitivity to pollutants, Chronic exhaustion, Epilepsy, Alzheimer

- Emotional Dysfunction: Depression, Obsessional thinking, Confusion

- Life Lesson: Selflessness

Goals: Expanded Consciousness

- Fears: Decision making

- Sutra to be Followed: Sutra of Allowing

•Positive Poles: Peace with self

•Too Open: Manic Depressive, Confused sexual expression, Frustration, Sense of unrealized strength

•Blocked: Constantly exhausted, Cannot make preference, No experience of belonging

•Balanced: Magnetic character, Achieves miracles in existence, Transcendent, At peace with self

•Motto: Pure Consciousness

THE SEVEN CHAKRAS OR ENERGY CENTERS PROVIDE A CLEAR MAP OF OUR REALITY AND SPIRITUAL EVOLUTION...

Technique on Chakras Unfolding (After the practices given above)

Sit on a mat, Rug or a clean sheet of fabric on the ground.. Spine straight away

Hand on thighs, palm open

Take a deep breath and lighten up… Do this for 3 times.. As you inhale and exhale feel the breath flowing all of your body..

Do opportunity respiratory, (Breath in from right nostril and breath out from left nostril and all once more breath in from left nose and breath out from right nose).. Do this for 10 times..

Now do the Energy burst exercising (Kapalbatti).. A hundred counts..

Relax for a while..

Now take a deep breath, Contract all of the muscle tissues of the perineum, keep the breath for 30 seconds, hobby on Moolaadhaar Chakra and launch the breath slowly..

During the rest way, respiratory must be deep.. Do this for 4 times..

Mentally chant the Beej mantra and recognition at the Chakra and you may experience the sensations and vibrations at the chakra going from base of the spine to the crown..

Now, Once yet again agreement all of the muscle mass of the perenium and preserve the breath for 1/2 of a minute and release.. Do this for four instances..

Continue the same for Swadhisthaan And Manipura..

At manipura chakra deliver your neck little upwards and chant outwardly the sound AA... For 7 times and then popularity on the chakra chanting the Beej Mantra..

Beej Mantras for all of the Chakras..

Moolaadhaar – Lam

Swadhishthaan – Vam

Manipuraka – Ram

Anahata – Yam

Vishuddhi – Hum

Agna – Aum

As you awareness on coronary coronary heart chakra revel in the increase and contraction of your chest.. Journey deep into your coronary

coronary heart and be there so long as you choice.. Keep chanting the Beej mantra alongside side your breath.. Now observe sandal paste on throat as Trishul Symbol (Half circle upwards with center finger and the middle line with shooting finger).. Breathe deeply as you chant the Beej Mantra.. Now bend your chin in order that it touches the middle of the collar bone and hold respiratory.. Be there for 3 minutes after which make you head ordinary and breathe from the throat.. Keep chanting the Beej Mantra.. Now bend your head backwards.. Bend as masses as possible (Do now not strain), Breathe from the center of eyebrows..

Now come all over again take the candle in your hands and hold it close to the Agna chakra simply so the heat is touched with the Chakra..(Lit the candle even as you start Vishuddhi, simply so Vishuddhi and Agna go with the flow collectively).. Chant the Beej Mantra AUM as loud as you can both from internal or outside..

Place the candle at the floor and notice the moderate from the Third Eye.. Be there as a whole lot as you may.. Feel the glide of your breath from the base of the backbone to the Top of your head.. (Sahasraar)..

Now get over again your reputation to Moolaadhaar see the moderate with all the gratitude in coronary heart and next hobby on Swadhisthaan, see the moderate with all of the gratitude in coronary heart and pass on upto Sahasraar..

Feel the sensations and vibrations all of your body and your self within the cocoon of moderate, Thank all the elements with all the gratitude from heart and slowly open your eyes..

All the on the same time as your workout Spine ought to be proper now and eyes closed..

Do the equal normal preferably within the early hours or evening amongst 5pm to 7pm..

Meditation and its Benefits

Meditation: enrichment on your soul

While the non secular benefit of meditation is exquisite bliss or enlightenment, those wards are not going to be understood as many… However, development inside the course of meditation and meditative techniques have several advantages at the gross frame or cloth level… It has been visible or shown that the advantages of meditation are more some distance-achieving and have a healing impact at the body and the mind… And also are available to you even as you're making meditation a everyday exercise of your lifestyles…

Body – Improvement of body lusture and massive fitness. When your mind focuses on a specific a part of the frame, the blood float to that difficulty will increase and cells get preserve of greater oxygen and different nutrients in abundance… Today, the numerous movie starts and fashion fashions include meditation of their every day regimen…

The maximum not unusual advantages that human body critiques due to meditation are as follows:

It allows in greater without issues falling asleep and snoozing soundly and moreover reduces sleep time…

It lowers oxygen consumption and decreases respiratory rate…

It will increase blood go with the flow and slows the coronary coronary heart charge developing the tolerance in coronary heart patients principal towards a deeper stage of relaxation… Brings B.P ordinary making particular for the patients with high blood stress…

Reduces anxiety attacks via reducing the stages of blood lactate…

Decreases muscle anxiety and complications… Builds self esteem and will growth serotonin manufacturing which impacts mood and behavior… Low tiers of serotonin are associated with despair, weight troubles, insomnia and complications…

Helps in continual diseases like hypersensitive reactions, arthritis and lots of others… Also reduces pre-menstrual syndrome and lets in in located up operative healing…

Enhances the immune device… Research has observed out that meditation will increase hobby of "natural-killer cells", which kill bacteria and maximum cancers cells… Also reduces interest of virus and emotional misery…

MIND:

Due to the busyness of life, our minds are regularly whole of conflicting thoughts and problems. Negative self speak impacts our attitudes and influences how we see the sector round us. Meditation clears the thoughts and improves the potential to pay attention making enjoy tons less forced and higher able to think actually.

A strong mind has manipulate over mind and moves and meditation facilitates to strengthen the mind. Many excessive profile people and sportsmen meditate regularly to enhance their performance. Nothing is better and less tough than meditation, close to resolving the problem of phobias.

Meditation can help a person expand a balanced and energetic character. Also allows in lowering careworn thinking, tension, tendency to worry, despair, tension, irritability and moodiness. Meditation additionally lets in in developing the ability to live calm in every scenario, will increase feelings of electricity, and enhances emotions of happiness and further emotional balance.

Intellect:

Improve creativity and concept- Through meditation; you could smooth your mind of energy ingesting idea clutter. When idea noise is at a minimum, you allow region for mind of creativity, and regularly come to be inspired thru unknown motives which I like to call endless mind. When creativity and notion strike, take movement, you will be surprised on the effects of your actions whilst performing on stimulated thoughts.

Increased cognizance- For art work or play, consciousness is constantly crucial to do your extraordinary. We all have the functionality to create big energy with focused electricity. So, through meditation, you can grade by grade enhance recognition so that you may have a more effect collectively along with your time whilst meditating, going for walks or having a laugh.

Increased self area

Improved analyzing functionality and memory

Developed intuition

Enhancement of self-self warranty

Faster choice making- With clearer and extra targeted wondering, your selection making abilities are alternatively advanced. This allows you cut to easy out via statistics and make sound choices.

Soul:

Peace of thoughts, emotional and intellectual detachment, heightened attention of the inner self, the capability to look interior, past the body, thoughts and character. Discovery of the energy and focus past the ego... Discovery of 1's actual being, achieving self focus and non secular awakening, facilitates living in the present 2d.

Inner peace, experiencing 'oneness', will boom the synchronicity on your lifestyles, allows preserve topics in attitude, offers peace of mind, happiness… Helps you discover your reason, improved self actualization, elevated compassion, growing knowledge, deeper expertise of self and others, brings body, mind, spirit in concord, deeper degree of spiritual relaxation, multiplied popularity of oneself, permits test forgiveness, adjustments attitude within the course of life.

Scientific elements of meditation – A studies

Relaxation- Relaxation can be described as a surely perceived state or response wherein a person feels comfort of hysteria or strain.

Meditation is one of the techniques of relaxation. Both rest and meditation have a intellectual in addition to a bodily size. They are believed not splendid to have useful effects at the mind, but also on the frame itself. Meditation may be used as a remedy to help relieve pressure in conditions which encompass coronary artery (coronary coronary coronary heart) illness, critical high blood pressure, anxiety headache, insomnia, allergies, immune deficiency, panic and lots of others.

The fundamentals of mind waves- Brain waves are generated with the resource of the building blocks of your mind – the individual cells referred to as neurons. Neurons communicate with each specific thru electric powered powered changes. We can truely see those electric powered expenses within the shape of thoughts waves as shown in an EEG (Electro-encephalogram).

Brain waves are measured in cycles in line with second (hertz; Hz is the fast form). We additionally talk approximately the 'frequency' of mind wave interest. The lower is the quantity of Hz, the slower is the mind interest or the slower is the frequency of the pastime. Researchers inside the 1930's and 40's indentified numerous special forms of mind waves. Traditionally, those fall into four types

Delta waves (Below 4Hz) upward push up throughout sleep.

Theta waves (four-7 Hz) are associated with sleep, deep rest, (like hypnotic relaxation), and visualization.

Alpha waves (8-thirteen Hz) occur whilst we're comfortable and calm.

Beta waves (13-38 Hz) rise up whilst we're actively thinking hassle-solving, and many others. There is one extra class it truly is

Gamma brain waves (39-one hundred Hz) are involved in better highbrow interest and consolidation of statistics. An interesting look at has proven that advanced Tibetan meditators produce higher levels of gamma than non meditators each before and in some unspecified time in the future of meditation.

We tend to count on we are generating one sort of thoughts wave. However those aren't clearly 'separate' mind waves – the sorts are simplest for consolation. They help describe the modifications we see in brain hobby for the duration of tremendous varieties of sports activities sports.

Early scientific research on the neuro-body shape or meditation focused on adjustments in mind wave (EEG) patterns, and variations in mind wave styles among meditators and non-meditators. In precis, meditation was proven to:

•Increase alpha (eight-13 Hz or cycles in line with 2d) production.

•Increase theta (4-7Hz) manufacturing.

•Increase excessive beta (20-40Hz) interest (with professional meditation)

Chapter 7: Causes For Diseases

Diagnosis has superior right into a notable art work in present day English medication. Thousands of lab checks, X-rays, ultrasound scans, and CT scans. Many contemporary-day strategies consisting of microscopes and MRI scans have been found to understand the reason of the disease and to diploma the man or woman of the sickness. Sometimes it's far said that the rate of the tests to discover what the sicknesses are greater than the charge of treating the ailment.

But irrespective of the deliver of many modern-day scientific gear, handiest the immediately purpose of a disease may be discovered in English treatment. Most of the time, the basis motive of the illness is unknown. Even in case you get at once remedy from the disorder, it isn't everlasting comfort from the ailment.

Why this deficiency in modern medicinal drug? Modern medication handiest examines and treats most effective the Physical frame.

Modern remedy does no longer recollect the 'Force' which activates the Physical frame.

There isn't any knowledge or clarity about them in technological statistics up to now.

Subtle global – (Sutchama World)

We recognize & diploma this worldwide and the universe via our five senses. But past our senses, there are three subtle worlds that are not able to apprehend with the aid of our senses. It is genuinely in the form of Energy.

• The life force within the frame

• Chakras that generate strength

• Nadis (Channels) that supply strength

• Energy our bodies for the duration of the frame

There is a subtle global existing in and round our physical frame. It can't be virtually measured through using way of senses or scientific gadgets.

However, our ancestors already determined severa hundred years inside the beyond with their information. Only with an facts of this diffused international of strength, we are capable of find out the idea reason of illnesses. It may be absolutely constant. This is in which contemporary English treatment fails. The understanding of our Siddhas / Ancestors/forefathers prevails!

Causes for any sickness will begin, exceptional from the subtle frame. (Exception – Accidents, injuries, Fire injuries, poisonous bites from bugs or animals, ingesting poison, etc.)

Three Bodies in Yoga: Sthula-Gross Body, Linga-Subtle Body & Karan-Causal Body - Fitsri

The Subtle Body is a combination of the Energy frame (Pranamaya Kosha), Emotional body(Manomaya Kosha), and Wisdom Body (Vinjanamaya Kosha).

Primarily all ailments are beginning in strength our bodies

If the ones defects in the strength our bodies, energy channels, or chakras are identified at an early diploma, they do now not alternate into illnesses. If we overlook about those defects, it'll increase. Above a quality degree, they come to be sicknesses.

Treating handiest the bodily frame (tablets, injections, and plenty of others.) can deliver a transient appearance of recuperation. But in a brief span of time, it's going to come all over again. Healing the Defects within the electricity our our bodies (correcting the inspiration motives) exceptional can prevent ordinary ailments and benefit everlasting treatment alternatives.

Our ancestors have listed 4 fundamental motives of defects in electricity our our bodies:

• Energy blockages/stagnation in electricity our our bodies.

• Defects inside the moves of the chakras.

• Blockages In electricity-carrying channels (Nadis)

• Disturbances in balancing the 5 Elements

(Panjabuthas) in our frame.

Why do defects rise up within the strength body, chakras, nadis, panchabhutas (Five Elements)? Our Siddhas / Ancestors have discovered the cause for the ones defects as well. They are listed beneath

• Negative thoughts and movements.

• Incorrect respiratory

• Improper meals behavior

• Improper existence.

After numerous years of research, Modern Medicine also accepts the above motives of illnesses. However, our Siddhas / Ancestors furnished the ones records through their understanding numerous loads of years in the past.

Impact of Negative mind

Negative wondering like anger, and hatred will cause peptic ulcer illness. Increases B.P., purpose coronary coronary heart diseases, and increases blood sugar stages. In mind

Negative thoughts that have collected in the thoughts over the years, cause most cancers.

Basic statistics approximately Mudra Therapy

MUDRAS

What is Mudra?

◉ Mudras are hand gestures used on the facet of pranayama (yogic respiratory sporting sports)

◉ Mudras act to stimulate taken into consideration certainly one of a kind components of the body concerned with respiration and to have an effect on the go together with the go together with the flow of electricity within the body or even one's temper.

◉ Mudras offer the energy same to complex yoga postures.

◉ Mudras Can be finished by using the use of Juniors to Seniors. No age guidelines to workout.

◉ This is "Boon for Elderly people", which they feel difficult in appearing complex Five palms on our hand constitute the ..." top="410" width="546">

Important Note approximately Mudra Therapy

●Mudra Therapy is not towards any other remedy plans.

●Mudra Therapy want to no longer be considered as an opportunity to medical treatments

●It is clearly useful to take Mudra treatment as a Supportive Therapy on the identical time as present process any scientific remedies.

●Follow your clinical clinical physician's recommendation and take your medicinal pills regularly.

●Reduce the severity of the disease through operating towards Mudras – regularly lessen consumption of drug remedies along with your physician's permission till the disease is absolutely cured.

●Even in case you sense it, are attempting to find advice out of your circle of relatives doctor/professional physician who's treating you.

●It's crucial to make certain diseases heal surely, after receiving confirmation out of your medical doctor.

●After that you could definitely prevent taking the medicine and capsules prescribed via your doctor.

●You must have a totally specific attention on the following whilst running in the direction of Mudras for chronic ailments which consist of

1. Diet

Once the feeding patterns are corrected, the energy of the diseases will lower extensively. Because 'Food is remedy. Have Natural meals, rather than poisonous, excessive ldl ldl cholesterol, Salty, Oily, Excess Sugar, Excess Sour, junk / packed food.

2. Water

Drink Water first-rate while you revel in thirsty. While eating water, chunk the water and swallow it slowly.

3. Body Workout

Have a practice of walking, doing asanas & pranayamas, or any smooth physical wearing activities. Because while we aren't giving any bodily interest to our body, it'll invite illnesses.

four. Rest & Sleep

It is so crucial to take proper sleep/relaxation just like bodily sports activities. You want to sleep a minimum of 6 hours and a most of 8 hours an afternoon.

five. Peaceful Mindset

Avoid terrible mind, Always Think honestly. Practice meditations to make yourself non violent.

Pre — Requisites in advance than starting Mudras

- Place

Practice Mudras on a Flat surface, with outstanding air circulate and colourful mild inside the room. (You can lie down in mattress as nicely at the identical time as working towards mudras however keep away from pillows)

- Time

After freshen-up inside the early morning, drink a tumbler of water and exercise mudras. It can be practiced within the morning, afternoon, nighttime, and night time time. Advised to exercise on an Empty Stomach for faster and preferred results. (three to 4 hours hole after having meals)

- Posture

You can sit in Padmasan, Suhasan, Vajrasan, in a chair, or mendacity at the mattress as properly. But ensure your Spine, Neck, and Head are immediately.

- Breathing

While running closer to Mudras, deep and normal respiration is crucial. No want to keep (Retention) your breath for a long time.

- Thought office work

Concentrate on the mudras and hobby on respiratory and the betterment of your health. Think awesome approximately your health. You can repeat excessive first-rate fitness affirmations at the equal time as training Mudras.

- Duration

Minimum 6 mins and Maximum 24 minutes. Some of the mudras want to be practiced for as lots as forty five minutes based totally absolutely clearly at the health requirements.

5 Stages in Curing Chronic Diseases

Stage 1: Removing the Toxins from the frame

Duration: 14 Days - 2 to 24 minutes

Stage 2: Balancing the Five Elements

Duration: 14 Days - 2 to 24 minutes

Stage 3: Balancing the Dasa Vayus (10 Gases)

Duration: 7 Days - 2 to 24 minutes

Stage four: Resolving Constipation

Duration: 2 to 24 mins (Stage three & 4 can practiced together)

Stage 5: Peaceful mind-set - Chin Mudra / Gyan Mudra

Duration: Every day Before Going to Bed 2 to 24 mins

Stage 6: Mudras for the health problems

Duration: Till it treatments virtually - 2 to 24 minutes

Stage 1: Detoxification

Stage 1: Detoxification

The waste products that live inside the body end up the cause of diseases. No man or woman can escape from this accumulation of waste products in the frame.

Before beginning the Mudras to hold health or cast off gift ailments, we are capable of now discover a smooth Mudra to first flush out the waste and pollution that have accumulated inside the frame for decades.

Procedure:

Gently contact the 0.33 digit of the ring finger with the quit of the thumb. Gentle stress is sufficient. Need to workout in each fingers with the aid of concentrated on everyday breathing.

Duration: 2 – 24 minutes

Benefits:

The wastages and pollutants that have been saved inside the body for a long term will go away slowly.

The body is probably cleansed and rejuvenated.

Diseases will depart.

Not simplest the dirt gathered in the frame however additionally the prevailing dirt will disappear

Stage 2: Balancing Five Elements

Stage 2: Balancing Five Elements

Everything in the universe is created thru the mixture of 5 Elements! There are Water, earth, air, sky, and fireplace are the five factors known as Pancha Buddhas. Our frame is made from panchabudhas and each tissue and organ of the body is whole of Panchabudhas.

If the proportions and ratio of the 5 elements in our frame are regular, we can be healthy.

Health Problems might also moreover moreover come whilst there are imbalances in the five elements.

There can be little imbalances in the 5 elements that seem in all of us's frame. However, it's going to healing itself. It is best while the ones deficiencies persist, above a awesome diploma continuously, then they grow to be sicknesses.

Deficiencies in the ones Panchabudhas have an impact at the frame's movements and purpose damage to the frame's internal organs.

Our Every finger will constitute each detail.

By folding, extending, and turning into a member of our arms, we are capable of carry out the balancing. To reduce, boom, lower and balance every detail, we've separate mudras. When we workout mudras for a selected detail, it is going to be SynchroMiss" top="363" width="283">

Chapter 8: Prithvi Mudra

Procedure:

Connect the Tip of the hoop finger and the thumb; the alternative 3 palms want to be straight. Need to exercise in each fingers with slight pressure through focused on ordinary respiratory.

Duration: minimal 2 – most 24 mins

Benefits:

The Air Element is probably balanced

The body turns into business enterprise

The energy degree of the frame rises.

Increases morale and self-self perception.

The body may want to have a modern-day glow.

Body and thoughts come to be slight.

Body temperature is balanced.

Decreases body weight.

Heaviness in the Body will disappear.

There is probably balance in existence.

Both body and thoughts are stopped from wandering and are available under our manage.

Clear considering existence and its purpose.

The thoughts will increase. Narrow-minded mind can also even disappear.

Patience will enlarge.

Increases hair increase with the resource of doing the topics taken efficaciously.

Fewer obstacles on the equal time as taking walks

Increase digestive power.

Dissolves phlegm, Cold, stuffy nostril, and frequent sneezing, Sinus may be managed

Varuna Mudra

Procedure:

Connect the Tip of the little finger and the thumb; the alternative three hands have to be without delay. Need to practice in each hands with mild strain with the useful resource of that specialize in ordinary respiratory.

Duration: minimal 2 – most 24 mins

Benefits:

Reduces body warmth. The texture of the pores and skin is vibrant.

Many pores and pores and skin illnesses will disappear.

The glide of strength inside the frame is easy.

The blood will thicken. Blood float is probably everyday. The

blocks within the blood float will disappear.

Swelling in feet and arms will disappear.

Thirst will lower.

Wrinkles at the pores and skin will disappear.

Reduces Laziness and lethargy in the body and mind and

makes energetic and active.

Makes to appearance extra younger

Menstrual troubles in women will disappear

Difficulty in urinating will decrease.

Reduces hair loss. Increases hair increase

Mucus, phlegm, and so on. Will lower.

Memory will increase.

Surya Mudra

Procedure:

Fold the hoop finger (fourth finger) and touch the zero.33

line under the thumb. Fold the thumb over the ring

finger (fourth finger) and have a examine little strain. The fantastic

3 fingers have to be right away.

Need to practice in each arms with gentle stress thru using

concentrated on regular respiration.

Duration: minimal 2 – most 24 minutes

Benefits:

Body warm temperature will increase.

The frame is business enterprise.

The frame becomes energetic.

Increases digestive power.

The coronary coronary heart becomes more potent. Heart ailments will

disappear.

Blood drift can be ordinary. Blockages and obstructions in

the blood float could be eliminated.

Phlegm will dissolve.

Reduces breathing illnesses.

Thyroid deficiency will disappear.

Increases intellectual balance.

Mental confusion will decrease.

Weight loss. The fat saved in the body dissolves.

Cholesterol degrees in the blood will lower.

Stage three: Balancing the Dasa Vayus (10 Gases)

7 Days

2 to 24 minutes

Balancing DasaVayus

So a protracted manner we've got discovered out Detoxification and five Element mudras. For any persistent sickness, it's far very critical to do the ones mudras earlier than beginning the mudra remedy for it.

The first degree of the remedy is to perform the Detoxification Mudras for 14 days continuously to flush out the crucial wastes and pollution which have collected in the frame.

The 2nd diploma of treatment is to correct the adjustments inside the regular u.S. Of the frame's panchabhuta Shaktis (Five Elements) thru the Five Element Mudras.

Chapter 9: Importance Of Ten Gases (Dasa Vayus)

Life Force

The Energy which gives and directs the existence inside our body is Life Force. When this Life Force electricity is healthy, the body and its movements are healthful. The changes in the level or incorrect movements of this crucial electricity cause illnesses.

When the actions of this Life Force are stopped, it outcomes in dying. When the Life Force power stops/leaves the body, the Soul will go away the body. Many human beings mistake lifestyles pressure and soul as one. These are extraordinary. Thus, existence stress may be very critical not pleasant for the movement of the body however additionally for the movement of the soul.

Other Names of Life Force:

This existence pressure is referred to through brilliant names in every america of the us of the us and in every way of life, for example,

• The British call this Life Force strength as Vital Energy.

• Dr. Hahnemann, hailed as the daddy of homeopathic treatment gave this lifestyles pressure a call: Elan Vitale.

• Biomagnetic Energy in Europe.

• Susputene, the daddy of Mesmerism, referred to Life Force as Animal Magnetism.

• Life energy is called Plasmic Energy thru Soviet scientists.

Ancient Chinese clinical texts communicate to this Life Force strength as Qi (or) Chi.

Our ancestors Named this life pressure as PRANA.

We can use the call given with the resource of way of our forefathers. PRANA moreover represents breathing air.

Based at the abilties of PRANA SAKTHI, it's far been divided into ten sub-divisions. These 10 sub-divisions can also be known as as Dasa Vayus (The 10 Gases).

DASA VAYUS

Sl.No Names Functionalities

1 Pranan - Respiration

2 Apanan - Excretion

three Vyanan - Circulation of blood

4 Udanan - Speech

5 Samanan - Digestion

6 Naagan - Vision

7 Koorman - Eyes

8 Girugaran - Sneezing

nine Devathathan - Yawning

10 Dhananjayan - Decomposition of the body after loss of existence gases)

1. Pranan

Pranan isn't always similar to Prana. Prana is the Life Force which consists of all of the 10 Gases. Pranan is a subdivision of the Life pressure known as Prana, which travels upward from the heart thru the nose. It has vital features.

●Creating starvation & thirst

●Digestion of food.

2. Apanan

Apanan stands in the course of the anus and genital organs and

controls their movements. It has essential functions:

• Excretion of wastes and urine.

• To ejaculate throughout sexual sex.

3. Vyanan

As it pervades all parts of the body, consequently it's far referred to as as

Vyanan: (pervasive).

The vital functionality of this Gas to revel in the feel

of touch (contact).

Another foremost function is to take the nutrients to the

cells in numerous elements of the body after the food is

digested.

3. Udanan

Udanan is placed inside the Throat location. Its maximum vital

functionality is speek and making a song •

Apart from this, Utanan makes our five senses to

take a rest even as drowsing, and after wide conscious; it resumes the

functionalities of the 5 senses.

five. Samanan

Samanan is located inside the Nabi (Belly button)region

Its obligation is to preserve the equilibrium of different

gases. Hence it is known as Samanan.

• Samanan is the gas that nourishes the frame.

6. Naagan

Naagan presents sight to our eyes

It stands on the throat causes vomiting and moreover motives snoring and laziness.

7. Koorman

Gas that operates the eyelids.

Opening and last the eyes, blinking.

Goosebumps, laughter, making the face glow and facial

expressions are managed by way of Koorman.

8. Girugaran

This fuel creates Sneezing. This fuel prevents germs such

as dirt, and bacteria virus that enters the nostril from outside

and enter the frame and purpose ailments.

If the Girugaran fuel is working flawlessly, it is able to prevent you via

developing sneezing, from airborne sickness moving into the

nostril. The not unusual airborne sicknesses are TB

(tuberculosis), Viral illnesses like influenza and anthrax,

and so on.

If Girugaran Vayu works nicely, such germs enter the nose

and reason a sneeze to expel them; Diseases do no longer rise up.

Air-borne illnesses can without troubles have an impact on people if the

Girukaran gasoline is not balanced of their our bodies.

9. Devadatta

Yawning and hiccups are every created through the use of the gas

Devadatta.

According to Science, yawning takes location while the mind

does no longer get sufficient Oxygen (Prana). When you yawn,

the stagnant carbon dioxide gasoline (Apana) is released and

the extra prana gasoline is drawn into the mind and it starts

strolling perfectly and disappears Fatigue. Devadatta fuel takes duty for entire thoughts functionalities.

10. Dhananjeyan

When life leaves the frame, the other 9 gases moreover go away the frame. But only this

Dhananjeyan Gas stays in the body for approximately three days. It reasons numerous chemical changes within the useless frame and reasons the frame to swell and decay. That's why we call it 'Decomposition fuel'. When the frame is cremated, this fuel comes out with the useful resource of the use of breaking the scalp. If the frame is buried, on the 0.33 day it's miles going out via the scalp.* Not handiest in dying. Dhananjeyan Vayu additionally plays a

very crucial feature in start. The critical feature of this Dhananjaya Vayu is to open the mother's cervix and push the toddler out as quickly because the fetus reaches its entire development diploma.

Prana Mudra:

The ring and little fingertips need to hook up with

the give up of the thumb with moderate stress on both fingers.

Remaining fingers want to be immediately.

Duration : 2 to 48 mins / day

Note: When doing this prana mudra, Mooladhara Chakra (first chakra) is inspired , strengthened and Increases its normal overall performance. Prana Shakti & Kundalini Shakthi has close connection to Mooladhara Chakra. When the Mooladhara is powerful, Prana Shakti will produce in abundance and additionally stimulates Kundali Shakti

Benefits:

Body and mind may be calm. The power of the body

will increase. The frame will become more potent.

Creates freshness and activeness.

Disappears Excessive delight and restlessness

Thinking becomes smooth.

Evil mind and negative thoughts within the thoughts will

disappear and offers you proper thoughts

Satisfies the mind.

Mental energy may even growth.

Provides you with specific preference-making energy.

Gives clarity on the reason of existence, and the dreams to be completed.

Selfishness will lower.

Spiritual inclination will growth.

Apana Mudra:

Procedure:

The ring and center fingertips need to connect to the stop

of the thumb with gentle strain on each arms.

The closing arms should be without delay.

Duration: 2 to 48 minutes/day

Chapter 10: The Heart Furthermore Gets Stronger

Fears and confusion inside the thoughts will disappear.

Increases morale.

Increases self-self perception.

Mind and wondering turn out to be smooth.

Eliminates Negative thoughts and Emotions, and fills with authentic thoughts.

Cures Constipation

Piles may be cured

Gastritis is probably cured.

Diabetes level is probably on pinnacle of things.

Kidneys and their system may be bolstered.

Cures Dental problems and strengthens enamel and gums.

Strengthens Stomach and Intestines.

The liver, Pancreas, Gall bladder, and Spleen is probably reinforced.

Strengthens breathing machine.

Excess warm temperature inside the body is probably removed through sweat.

Makes Menstrual cycles regular and stops greater

bleeding.

Improves Potency. Resolves sexual problems.

Helps Normal Delivery.

Note: Don't Practice Apana Mudra, at the same time as you are having

vomiting and diarrhea.

Udana Mudra:

Procedure:

The index, middle, and ring fingertips want to attach

with the pinnacle of the thumb with mild strain on every fingers.

The closing little finger want to be instantly.

Duration: 2 to 24 mins/day

Benefits

Udana mudra advantages the vocal cords (voice), the

respiration device, and the thyroid-parathyroid glands.

The parathyroid gland is on pinnacle of things of the kidneys.

With this mudra, the parathyroid gland skills well, and kidney troubles are solved.

The speech becomes clean.

The breathing device works higher.

Limbs get power and that they turn out to be strong

Vyana Mudra:

Procedure:

The index and middle finger suggestions need to connect with tip of the thumb with slight pressure in each hands.

Remaining palms should be proper now.

Duration: 2 to 24 minutes / day

Benefits

It maintains the Blood Pressure in normal degree.

Reduces the body pain because of the Vayu Dosha.

Improves the power and sports of all Nadis

(Channels).

It gets rid of fatigue, laziness, dizziness.

Resolves General weak spot due to much less sleep.

Improves Mental Stability.

Provides Zeal, freshness to thoughts, liveliness to the

body

Functioning of coronary coronary heart can be progressed.

It offers ideal manage over excessive sweating.

Samana Mudra:

Procedure:

All the pointers of the arms need to connect with moderate

stress in each hands.

Duration: 2 to 24 mins / day

Benefits

Increases Samana Vayu.

Balances all of the 10 Gases (Dasa Vayus)

Nutrients in food are surely damaged down and

transported at some point of the body through the blood.

Improves frame growth

Actions in Subtle frame come to be everyday.

Internal organs is probably bolstered.

Strengthens thoughts, Evil mind and bad emotions

will disappear and the mind becomes clear.

Good thoughts and thoughts might be shaped.

Increases the strength diploma in the body.

Panchabhutas (Five Elements) may be balanced

Stage four: Resolving Constipation

2 to 24 minutes

(Stages three & four can be practiced collectively)

Note:

It may be very critical for humans with constipation

issues to get it regular in advance than starting remedy for any

ailment. This applies not handiest to mudra remedy however

additionally to allopathic, Marma, Siddha, Ayurveda,

Homeopathy, and so forth.

Mudras for Constipation

Sooji Mudra and Mushti Mudra both treatment constipation. Making some adjustments in the weight loss program and way of life, the ones Mudras can supply greater benefits.

Sooji Mudra:

Procedure:

Clench every hands and wrap them up collectively together with your thumb All four hands need to be folded tightly with the thumb placed over the middle finger. Keep the Mudra near the chest, slowly bypass the right hand to the right aspect and the left hand to the left aspect (in a tightly closed feature) and expand the index fingers (stretch) in each palms while slowly breathing in. While you exhale, fold the index finger alongside side the opposite palms and bring it straight away to the chest. Keep the entire attention on the Mudra. (Extending the index finger whilst inhaling and folding all of the fingers within the route of exhale is one cycle)

Duration: 8 to 23 cycles/day

Benefits

Constipation will disappear

If you try this mudra every day, accrued waste products

and toxins inside the frame can be cleansed.

People who take drug remedies for ailments for an prolonged period

of time have more residues of their frame. These residues

also are poisonous materials. These also can cause the

improvement of many new illnesses. These wastes are

additionally expelled from the body even as sooji mudra is

practiced constantly.

A character tormented by Migraine, Sinus, Asthma,

Allergy, Skin Disease, Stomach, Intestinal Disease and masses of others., if

he practices this mudra every day, the depth of the contamination

can be decreased substantially.

Mushti Mudra:

Procedure

All four hands have to be folded tightly and the top of

thumb must touch the ring finger. Hold the mudra in

each arms. Concentrate on the Mudras and respiratory.

Duration: 2 to 24 mins / day

Benefits:

Constipation will disappear

Improves digestive energy

Increases urge for meals.

Increases self-self perception and braveness.

Stage five: Peaceful thoughts-set

 Chin Mudra / Gyan Mudra Before Going to Bed

2 to 24 mins

Mudra for Peaceful Mindset

Chin / Gyan Mudra

Procedure

Tip of the index and thumb want to be joined, the very last

three hands should be right now. Hold the Mudras in Both

fingers thru way of making use of slight stress and observe the

breathing.

Duration: 2 to 24 minutes/day

Benefits:

Mind and thinking can be targeted.

Mind wandering will disappear.

The horrible mind and dirty thoughts that stay in

the thoughts and mind might be cleansed.

Anger, agitation, impatience, obstinacy, and so on. Will

disappear and a peaceful temper will growth.

There is probably readability in thoughts.

Fears will disappear.

Increases memory.

Self-self guarantee will growth.

The mind is actively superior mind functionality

The apprehensive system turns into robust.

Interest in studying and mastering will growth.

Mudra permits students lots.

Chapter 11: Stress, Depression, And Depression May Step By Step Go

away.

Creativity and imagination frequently boom.

'Enquiry of Wisdom' will upward thrust up within the mind.

This "mudra of records" is the first step at the direction to enlightenment

Stage 6: Mudras for health problems

2 to 24 mins

Mudras for Health Issues (Healing Mudras)

Padma / Pankaja Mudra – Strengthens Nervous System

Procedure

At first, make Namaste Posture by manner of turning into a member of the 2 arms

Then be a part of the guidelines of each little palms component thru aspect. Likewise, connect the recommendations of every thumbs, aspect via the use of aspect. Wrists in

every palms must be joined at the wrist and the opposite

palms should be straight away. Contracting and increasing

the hands is one cycle.

Duration: Minimum 10 cycles and most 23 cycles.

Benefits:

Strengthens Nervous System

Reduces Excessive frame warm temperature

Protects the heart

Strengthens backbone

Provides you staying power

Maintains regular body warm temperature.

Linga Mudra – Cold / Sinus / Immunity Power

Procedure:

First through the nostrils inhale and exhale very slowly.

Then be part of both arms and hold nice the left thumb

upright and keep all of the fantastic hands connect with each other as validated within the image. Perform the vice-versa for each other thumb as nicely.

Duration: 2 mins to 24 mins.

Benefits

Cure Cold / Sinus.

Increases immunity strength

Strengthens lungs

Will lessen extra body weight

Aadhi Mudra – balances Life Force , Bright Thoughts , Immunity Power, Peace of Mind

Procedure:

Place your thumbs in each palms and cover the

thumb with the closing four palms with employer pressure.

Hold this mudra in each hands.

Duration: 2 minutes to 24 minutes

Benefits:

Balances Life Force

Brings Bright Thoughts

Provides Immunity Power,

Gives peace of Mind

Activeness at some point of the day

Gives enthusiasm

Rudra Mudra – Piles, Hernia, Stomach Related issues, Uterus Strengthening

Procedure:

Connect the give up of the thumb with suggestions of the index and

ring finger, final two arms want to be proper now.

Hold this mudra in each palms.

Duration: 2 mins to 24 mins

Benefits:

Cures Piles & Hernia

Stomach associated troubles may be resolved

Strengthens Uterus

Hakkini Mudra – Good Concentration, Memory, Refreshes Brain – Best for Students

Procedure:

Connect the guidelines of all the arms in each fingers with a

mild stress.

Duration: 2 minutes to 24 minutes

Benefits:

Gives properly cognizance.

Improves memory energy.

Refreshes brain cells.

Beneficial mudra for college students

Anusasana Mudra – Strengthens Spinal Cord, Back Pain & Neck Pain

Procedure:

Fold the center finger, ring, and little finger and call the inner aspect of the palm, cover the three folded palms

at the side of your thumb. Make the index finger right away.

Duration: 2 mins to 24 mins

Benefits:

Strengthens spinal twine.

Resolves back pain.

Resolves neck pain.

Shankh Mudra – Throat Problems, Stammering

Procedure: Place the left thumb at the right palm; now cowl the

left thumb with 4 hands in the right hand.

Now deliver four arms inside the left palm and vicinity on top

of the 4 palms in the proper hand.

Join the top of the proper thumb with 4 hands from the

left hand as verified in the photo. Do the Vice-Versa (for

some different hand as well).

Duration: 2 mins to 24 mins.

Benefits:

All troubles in Throat is probably cured

Stammering can be cured.

Thyroid degree turns into everyday.

Will get Soothing Voice

Strengthens the Uterus.

Strengthens Zygote and permits the toddler boom inside the womb.

Resolves impotency for every men and women.

Surabhi Mudra – Rheumatoid Arthritis

Procedure:

Connect the right little finger with the left ring finger.

Connect the proper ring finger with the left little finger.

Connect the right index finger with the left middle finger.

Connect the proper middle finger with the left index finger.

Stretch the thumb in each fingers.

Duration: 2 to 24 minutes

Benefits:

Cures Rheumatoid Arthritis and Cures Autoimmune sicknesses

Spine / Back Mudra – Back Pain, Hip Pain, Strengthens Kidney, Small & Large Intestine, Lungs, Heart, Liver, Spleen, Pancreas

Procedure:

Connect the index and thumb within the left hand, the final 3 fingers need to be right now. Connect the tips of the center, little, and thumb hands within the right hand, the remaining index and ring arms want to be instantly.

Duration: 2 to 24 minutes

Benefits:

Resolves Back Pain

Resolves Hip Pain

Strengthens Kidney

Strengthens Small & Large Intestine

Strengthens all of the King Organs - Lungs, Heart, Liver,

Spleen & Pancreas.

Prana Mudra – Sharp Eyes, Immunity Power, Prana Energy

Procedure: The ring and little fingertips need to connect with the surrender of the thumb with mild pressure on each hands.

The last fingers should be right away.

Duration: 2 to forty eight mins/day

Benefits:

Body and mind might be calm. The electricity of the frame

will boom. The frame turns into more potent.

Creates freshness and activeness.

Disappears Excessive pride and restlessness

Thinking becomes easy.

Evil mind and poor thoughts inside the thoughts will

disappear and offers you suitable thoughts

Satisfies the thoughts.

Mental electricity may additionally even growth.

Chapter 12: The Ring And Center Fingertips Want To Hook Up With Tip

of the thumb with slight pressure in each hands.

Remaining palms should be immediately.

Duration: 2 to forty eight mins/day

Benefits:

Eliminates the accrued waste products inside the body

Through sweat, feces and urine. It purifies the body.

Diseases due to the buildup of waste products

can be cured.

The body is active and strong.

The electricity stage of the frame will upward thrust

The nerves is probably robust.

The coronary heart moreover receives stronger

Fears and confusions in the thoughts will disappear.

Increases morale.

Increases self-self warranty.

Mind and wondering end up clean.

Eliminates Negative mind and Emotions, fills with

actual thoughts.

Cures Constipation & Gastritis

Piles can be cured

Diabetes level is probably in control.

Kidneys and the Kidney device can be strengthened.

Cures Dental issues and strengthens enamel and gums.

Strengthens Stomach and Intestines.

The liver, Pancreas, Gall bladder, and Spleen may be

bolstered.

Strengthens respiration tool.

Excess warmth within the body may be eliminated through sweat.

Makes Menstrual cycles everyday and forestalls extra

bleeding.

Improves Potency. Resolves sexual issues.

Helps Normal Delivery.

Note: Don't Practice Apana Mudra, on the identical time as you are having

vomiting and diarrhea.

Apana Vayu Mudra – Mudra for Heart – Heart Diseases, Chest Pain

Procedure:

Fold the index finger and contact the inner aspect of the

palm, ring and middle fingertips need to hook up with the pinnacle of the thumb with mild pressure in each hands.

The very last little finger ought to be proper now.

Duration: 2 to 48 minutes/day

Benefits:

This is Mudra for the Heart

Cure all Heart Diseases

Resolves Gastritis

Cures Chest Pain

Strengthens heart functionalities.

Asthma Mudra – Wheezing, Breathing Problems

Procedure:

Fold the center finger as an entire lot because the first digit in every fingers.

The final fingers ought to be straight away.

Duration: 2 to 48 mins/day

Benefits:

Asthma sickness may be on pinnacle of factors

Provides on the spot comfort from Wheezing, Breathing Problems

Practicing on regular basis can remedy Asthma honestly.

Swasa Kosha Mudra – Strengthens Respiratory System

Procedure:

Fold the little finger and permit the quit of the little finger to

contact the final digit (line) of the thumb,

Fold the hoop finger and permit the give up of the hoop finger contact

the number one digit (line) of the thumb.

Fold the center finger and allow the end of the middle finger

touch the stop of the thumb.

Let the index finger be instantly.

Duration: 2 to 48 minutes/day

Benefits:

Strengthens the Energy Body – Pranamaya Kosha

Strengthens the respiratory gadget.

Cures Lungs infections.

Cures all respiratory problems.

Bramara Mudra – Allergies

Procedure:

Fold the index finger and keep it in the base of the

thumb.

Extend the center finger and join the pinnacle of the

thumb with the sides of the middle finger.

Let the hoop and little palms are right away.

Fold the index finger and hold it within the base of the

thumb.

Extend the middle finger and be a part of the pinnacle of the

thumb with the rims of the middle finger.

Let the ring and little palms are right away.

Duration: 2 to forty eight minutes/day

Benefits:

Cures all allergic reactions (Dust, pollen, food, skin, and plenty of others).

Cures all respiration issues.

Udana Mudra – Improves Speech,O2 stage, Strengthens throat, Happiness

Procedure: Connect the index, center, and ring arms with the quit of the thumb. The little finger ought to be immediately.

Duration: 2 to 24 minutes

Benefits:

Improves Speech

Increases Oxygen diploma

Strengthens throat

Increases Happiness

Maha Siras Mudra – All Headaches, Peenisam, Sinus, Nose associated problems.

Procedure:

Connect the index, middle with tip of the thumb. Fold the

ring finger and speak to the inner facet of the palm. Little

finger must be right away.

Duration : 2 to 24 minutes

Benefits:

Cures every type issues in and spherical head.

Cures all kinds of Headaches,

Cures Peenisam (Kind of allergy inside the nose)

Cures Sinus

Resolves Nose related issues

Surya Mudra – Weight Loss, Controlling Thyroid

Procedure:

Fold the ring finger (fourth finger) and make contact with the 1/3

line beneath the thumb. Fold the thumb over the hoop

finger (fourth finger) and exercise little pressure. The splendid

three arms should be straight.

Need to practice in each arms with slight stress via

targeting regular respiration.

Duration: minimal 2 – maximum 24 minutes

Benefits:

Increases Body warm temperature.

The frame will become organisation and active.

Increases digestive energy.

The coronary heart becomes more potent. Heart illnesses will disappear.

Blood drift might be regular. Blockages and obstructions within the blood flow can be eliminated.

Phlegm will dissolve.

Reduces respiratory diseases.

Thyroid deficiency will disappear.

Increases intellectual stability.

Mental confusions will lower.

Weight loss. The fats saved within the frame dissolves.

Cholesterol tiers inside the blood will lower.

Joint (Mootu) Mudra – Pain in All the Joints 6 months

Procedure:

Connect the guidelines of the center finger and thumb in the left hand. Connect the tips of the hoop finger and thumb in the left hand. Remaining fingers in each palms need to be strainght.

Duration : 2 to 24 mins

Benefits:

Resolves pain in All the Joints

Ganesha Mudra – Strengthens Lungs & Heart

Ganesa Mudra - a easy mudra done through becoming a member of each

hands. Ganesha is taken into consideration because the remover of

obstacles and obstructions. This mudra is also removes

many miseries. That is why it's miles known as 'Ganesha Mudra'

after the decision of Ganesha who solves all of the problems

Procedure:

The left palm need to right away to the chest and

Palm handling outward. Bring the right palm coping with inwards

and Fold the palms of every fingers slightly and draw near

the hands of the left hand with the arms of the right

hand. Like a hook.

Now Exhale surely and tighten those hands.

Let the palms be right now to the chest Feel the tightness within the palms, muscle tissue inside the neck and rib region. Hold the retention breath for a few seconds then slowly inhale and launch the arms. Repeat this method for 6 instances.

After 2 mins rest, do the vice-versa and repeat it for 6

instances. After doing this mudra for 12 (6+6) instances, take some rest (Santhi Asana or Savasana) via lying down in a

mat. While doing this mudra, the spinal twine need to be

right now without bending.

It is critical that your complete hobby is centered on the mudra you're training.

Seating Pattern:

It is recommended to do Ganesa mudra at the identical time as reputation.

People who are not able to stand, can also do thru the usage of sitting.

People who are bedridden can do that mudra with lying

on mattress.

Benefits

Removes all obstacles and obstructions in lifestyles.

Cures Asthma

Makes the respiratory clean.

Strengthens coronary coronary heart and coronary heart associated functionalities.

Increases Self Confidence.

Reduces inferiority complex.

Anjali Mudra – Balances the Energy degree, Peace, Brain, Normal BP

Procedure:

Join every right and left hands on the facet of hands in each

hands and make Namaste (Wishing) Posture in the the front of

the chest.

Duration: 2 to 24 mins

Benefits:

Balances the Energy degree

Generates Peace

Improves the capability of Brain

156

Maintains Normal BP

Sumana Mudra – Liver, Gall Bladder, Nervous System, Heart, Diabetes

Procedure: Join the outer aspects hands of the left and right hand.

Make fine nails of the each hands are touching every

one-of-a-kind. Hold this Mudra in the front of the chest.

Duration: 2 to 24 minutes

Benefits:

Strengthens Liver, Gall Bladder

Strengthens Nervous gadget

Strengthens Heart and its functionalities.

Cures the diabetes.

Dhyana Mudra – Mind Relaxing, Meditation

Procedure:

Place the left palm on the middle of the Lower belly,

keep the proper palm on top of the left palm and feature a have a take a look at

the respiratory.

Duration: 2 to 24 mins

Benefits

Relaxes Mind

Useful for doing Meditation

Sivalinga Mudra – Body Mind & Soul, Spreads Positive Energy

Procedure:

Stretch the little and ring hands in both hands and be a part of every precise. Extend center and index palms and contact every different. Let the Thumb be part of around the palms.

Chapter 13: Swelling Within The Legs Because Of Extra Water Diploma Can Be

resolved.

One of the great mudra for resolving fitness troubles for ladies.

Moothrashaya Mudra — Kidney, Throat pain, Watery eyes, Eliminate bad water from the frame.

Procedure: Fold the hoop and little finger and cowl those palms with thumb in both arms. Let the opposite arms strethced as confirmed in the picture.

Duration: 2 to 24 minutes

Benefits:

All Kidney problems, Throat pain, Watery eyes may be resolved.

Swelling in the legs due to more water diploma can be

resolved.

Prasanna Mudra – Stops Hair loss, Normalize frame warmth

Procedure: Fold all of the fingers upto the primary digit (Let the nails and inner arms touch every one-of-a-type. Let the Thumb stretch and face the sky as demonstrated within the photograph.

Duration: 2 to 24 mins

Benefits:

Stops Hair loss

Normalizes body warmth

Pooshan Mudra – Digestive Power, Immunity strength, Universal Health (Left hand Apana, Right Vyana)

Procedure: Hold Apana mudra in Left hand Apana and vyana mudra in Right hand as shown in the image.

Duration: 2 to 24 minutes

Benefits:

Increases Digestive Power,

Increases Immunity power

Mudra for Universal Health

Usha Mudra – Impotency Both Men & Women, Reproductive Organs

Procedure: Cross all of the hands and be part of together in every palms as validated inside the photograph.

Duration: 2 to 24 minutes

Benefits:

Resolves impotency for Both Men & Women,

Strengthens Reproductive Organs

Easy for manifesting goals.

Aswini Mudra – Skin, Cancer, Activates Kundalini, Positive Thoughts, Discipline for Students

Procedure: Slowly Shrink the Anus and launch the Anus & Inhale. This is one cycle.

Duration: minimum 10 maximum 23 cycles.

Benefits

Resolves Skin troubles,

Destroys Cancer cells

Activates Kundalini shakthi,

Increases Positive Thoughts,

Gives field and true conduct for Students

Uthirapodhi Mudra – Strengthens Mind, Agility, Removes fear and undesirable

Procedure:

Cross the little, ring and center fingers in each palms and be part of together. Extend the index and thumb fingers and be a part of the suggestions of each finger. Keep the mudra infront of the chest and touch the tips of the thumb with middle of the chest rib. Face the index arms towards upward path.

Duration: 2 to 24 minutes

Benefits:

Strengthens Mind

Increases Agility

Removes fear and unwanted

Yoni Mudra – Strengthens Uterus, Heals all of the issues for the ladies at some stage in menopause

Procedure:

Interjoin the middle, ring and little hands in each palms. Connect and Extend the index and thumb palms as demonstrated in the icture.

Duration: 2 to 24 minutes

Benefits:

Strengthens Uterus,

Heals all of the problems for the girls during menopause

Kubera Mudra – Mudra for Wealth, Good Memory & Confidence

Procedure:

Join the pointers of index and middle fingers with tip of the thumb, fold the hoop and little palms to the touch the innerside of the palm.

Connect and Extend the index and thumb fingers as confirmed within the photo.

Duration: 2 to 24 mins

Benefits:

Mudra for Wealth

Good Memory & Confidence

eight.

Best Practices

Practice the Mudras within the early morning in empty

belly.

Practice mudras in advance than two hours of having food.

Concentrate on respiration at the same time as retaining mudras.

Visualize the better health whilst preserving mudras.

nine.

Testimonials

Mudras for General Practice:

 Category

 Mudras

Students

 Hakkini Mudra, Aadhi Mudra, Chin Mudra, Surya Mudra

Women

 Chin Mudra, Akasha Mudra, Surya Mudra, Madhangi Mudra, Yoni Mudra

Married Men

 Aadhi Mudra, Varuna Mudra, Vayu Mudra, Mugula Mudra

Diabetes

 Apana mudra, Varuna Mudra, Sumana Mudra, Chin Mudra

BP

 Aadhi Mudra, Chin Mudra, Shangh Mudra

Neck Pain

 Surya Mudra, Vayu Mudra, Anusasana Mudra

Thyroid

 Surya Mudra, Aadhi Mudra, Mugula Mudra

Menstrual troubles

 Akasha Mudra, Surya Mudra, Maadhangi Mudra, Yoni Mudra

Joint Pains

 Vayu Mudra, Apana Mudra, Apana Vayu Mudra, Joint Mudra, Mugula Mudra

Eye Diseases

 Prana Mudra , Linga Mudra , Mugula Mudra

Hair Fall

 Prasanna Mudra, Mugula Mudra, Maadhangi Mudra

14: The Basics

For the very first financial disaster of this e-book, it might be a fantastic concept to enlighten you with the basics approximately what Mudras truly are, and what they involve.

After all, in case you really need to have a smooth and strong expertise approximately something, it's miles essential to be nicely informed about the fundamentals.

It's like building a constructing—the more potent the lowest is, the sturdier the constructing can be.

This financial disaster goes to create the inspiration, upon which we can maintain to construct an great constructing of information.

What are Mudras?

'Mudra' is the Sanskrit phrase for 'mark' or 'seal'.

Mudras are, in short, any positions of your frame which have an impact at the energies of your body or your modern mood. While it is real that any a part of the body may be concerned in Mudras, it's also the hands and the palms which can be held in those specific positions.

IMPORTANT TO REMEMBER: We will study specifically Hand Mudras, however the fact that there are others the usage of exquisite frame factors. The Word Mudra on this e-book is used concerning Hand gestures.

Mudras are often finished even as one meditates. These positions had been used inside the Eastern Countries for hundreds of years, specially amongst cultures of Buddhism. Something you may have noticed is that many statues of Buddha will be inclined to reveal his arms held in a extremely good characteristic— the ones are Mudras used to assist on the journey to enlightenment. That is one of the reasons why humans use those positions to these days, notwithstanding the fact that a huge a part of practitioners use them for added direct advantages as we are able to have a look at in the direction of the e book.

Some of the most famous Mudras positions include sitting collectively together with your legs crossed, and putting your palms upon your knees in conjunction with your index arms touching the tips of your thumbs.

Besides to being used for meditation, Mudras have additionally been used in the past to deal with physical troubles collectively with cramps, dizziness and extra immoderate troubles, further to highbrow ailments consisting of anxiety or despair, for instance.

According to the philosophy that many people stand with the resource of, the bodily frame is crafted from five factors, each of them associated with a finger:

• Fire- Represented with the aid of using the Thumb

• Air- Represented via the Index finger

• Aakash(Sky and Space detail)- Represented by using the use of the Middle finger

• Earth- Represented by means of the usage of the Ring finger

• Water - Represented with the useful resource of the Little finger

Lack of right balance between those factors is what motives problems inside the frame and thoughts.

It is believed that plenty of those issues may be solved, consequently, with the useful resource of connecting positive additives of the body with Mudras.

The turning into a member of of great palms with others is executed to create a positive effect at the human body with the useful resource of purifying it and protective it from terrible forces.

That sums up the easy idea of what Mudras consists of.

Chapter 15: Birth Of Mudras

Mudras had been used for years upon years, but many people which may be interested by virtually making use of Mudras are unaware of their origins, and the way they came to be after which superior to come to be what they will be today.

In this bankruptcy, we're going to take a look at the fundamentals approximately the starting vicinity, records and improvement of Mudras. The motive to recognise about this information is just so it isn't always virtually an outside gesture that you carry out, but a symbol with a deeper meaning inside the back of it and a information that you are very well privy to. This manner, the Mudra ought to probable make more experience.

Only even as you realise those objects are you able to truly advantage all of the spiritual benefits of the usage of Mudras (hand Mudras) to your practices.

ORIGINS AND DEVELOPMENT

The origins of Mudras (which means any shape of body role, no longer first-class arms) date again to prehistoric times, even earlier than historic Eastern and Egyptian civilizations had been created. When the early civilizations started out out to enlarge, many photographs of gods and goddesses have been created which confirmed them sitting or reputation in some positions and preserving their palms out in a particular manner, i.E. Mudras.

As multiple religions started out to unfold across the world, some of the extra ultra-modern philosophies still protected Mudras into their traditions, celebrations, meditations, and so forth. In India, for instance, Mudras were applied in conventional dances, in addition to to "open" their thoughts and connecting with the superior strain or do away with stress from one's life. These hand gestures grew in importance for its effectiveness and additional people commenced out to recognize about them, coming across new ones and enhancing the older ones.

As stated earlier, Mudras specifically contain the hands, however there are wonderful ones which might be finished with different components of the body, permitting the power to go along with the float quicker and extra harmoniously in the body.

HISTORY OF WELL-KNOWN MUDRAS

Let's in brief see the records of a number of the famous Mudras. These Mudras were studied for loads of years as many sculptures and essential pictures show a number of them.

• The Abhaya Mudra, in which the open palm faces outward, is one of the most well known Mudras. It is concept to be originated from the depictions of Buddha, supposedly while he have turn out to be calming an elephant that attacked him (2500 years in the past about)

The starting area of this Mudra is what reasons human beings to partner it with peace, kindness and protection, and it is concept to have the capability to remove all your worry on the same time as used often.

In Thailand and some other areas, Abhaya Mudra is related with the taking walks Buddha, who is every so often tested appearing the Mudra uniformly with every palms.

• The Bhumisparsa or 'earth touching' Mudra is likewise a broadly identified one which originated from while Buddha took the earth as testimony after he had solved the issue of all human struggling at the identical time as he sat underneath a tree.

This Mudra is performed via putting the proper hand upon the right knee and pressing all the hands to the ground, maintaining the left hand flat in the lap.

• The Dharmachakra Mudra (written in Sanskrit) originated from a number one 2d in Buddha's life—even as he gave his first sermon after being enlightened, in Sarnath (a city positioned thirteen km away from Varnasi near the confluence of Ganges and Gomati rivers in Uttar Pradesh, India). During the 1/3 century B.C.

This Mudra is meant to symbolize the turning of the "wheel of the Dharma"— image representing the Dharma (or faith) in Hinduism, Buddhism and Jainism.

As an instance, high quality figures from Japan have furthermore been shown to be appearing this Mudra even earlier than the ninth century.

• The Dhyana Mudra originated from representations of Buddha, in addition to Amitabha (the important Buddha in Pure Land Buddhism, a department of East Asian Buddhism). It likely originated in the u . S . We in recent times understand as India and in China sooner or later of the Wei era. Wei technology. (386-534 A.D.) This Mudra is finished through placing the proper give up the left hand each facing upward, then joining the recommendations of thumbs from each fingers.

This Mudra has been used for restoration, enhancing attention similarly to for mediation.

• The Varada Mudra originated in China throughout the Wei length and in Japan within the path of the Asuka length (538-710 A.D.).

This Mudra modified into continuously paired with some exceptional Mudra however. Representing the "supplying a present" photo as visible on the image. Symbolizes the charity, the welcoming, compassion and sincerity.

In the Varada Mudra, the arm is crooked, the palm grew to end up up and the arms barely bent. At the begin, the hands had been stiff, but their function on this Mudra step by step commenced out to loosen, step by step the Mudra developed in order that the hands were surely curved.

These are only some of the maximum famous Mudras. As you now comprehend, they all have a wealthy records at the back of them (and we ought to bypass plenty deeper), originated and developed in lots of special techniques.

Chapter 16: Chakras And Mudras

Let's see what a Chakra is, and the distinctive styles of them—this bankruptcy will offer you with all the crucial information that you want to recognize approximately Chakras, and the way you could rent them in the precise way. In addition, we'll talk the relationship amongst Chakras and Mudras so you can understand how the 2 subjects supplement each specific and paintings in harmony to create powerful and effective outcomes.

WHAT ARE CHAKRAS?

The Sanskrit word for Chakra truely interprets to 'wheel'. When it consists of Yoga, this is meant to represent the wheels of strength which is probably found in our our our bodies. Think of it this way—there may be a spinning wheel of power in the vicinity wherein be counted range meets interest.

The strength that propels Chakras is the critical existence pressure, it's miles critical to hold us healthy and alive. Every Chakra consists of bundles of nerves similarly to our intellectual, emotional and spiritual united states of being.

That is the motive why preserving them opened, aligned and fluid is essential for feeling in a terrific mood.

In quick, a Chakra is a concept that includes seven facilities of spiritual power inside the human body.

TYPES OF CHAKRAS

meditation-1-1236900-1598x1103

Picture 1. Representation of the 7 Chakras.

There are seven specific styles of Chakras which you need to recognise approximately. We'll see them from the lowest of the backbone, to the pinnacle of the pinnacle (crown).

-The first Chakra is the Muladhara, this is the Chakra of balance, protection and our essential desires. It is present inside the first three vertebrae, the colon further to the bladder. Placed many of the anus and genital area. You can "open" this Chakra for feeling with extra energy and stable.

-Next, the Svadhisthana Chakra is the creativity middle, further to the sexual center. It is gift in the pubic bone and offers you with progressive topics, art, track, and masses of others.

-The 1/three Chakra is Manipura Chakra translates to "radiant gem", and it is gift inside the vicinity from the breastbone to the navel. This chakra is what gives us with our private power.

When you set up a enterprise agency maintain near in your first 3 chakras, which might be the bodily chakras, simplest then can you operate the non secular Chakras to their complete amount.

-The fourth Chakra is placed on the middle of the coronary coronary heart, and it unites all the chakras which is probably above and under it. This Chakra is also stated to behave as a bridge between our frame and our thoughts, and it's also our supply of compassion and love.ç

-The 5th Chakra is the Vishuddha Chakra, which gives us verbal expression and the power to talk the reality. This Chakra is gift inside the neck, mouth, tongue, thyroid, and plenty of others

-Next, the Ajna Chakra is gift proper among your eyebrows. It is what gives us with the mysterious experience called intuition.

-Lastly, the Sahaswara chakra is present on the crown of the head and is the chakra of enlightenment, the simplest representing the right to "recognize" and analyze extra from the area and our life. This Chakra has control over the rest.

OPENING CHAKRAS WITH MUDRAS

This section is all approximately learning the connection among Chakras and Mudras and the way we're capable of spark off Chakras.

The manner wherein Chakras and Mudras are associated is this:

Chakras may be 'opened' with the help of Mudras. Certain Mudras set off a few Chakras via funneling the energy in the direction of a few frame parts. We will see a way to activate the 7 Chakras the usage of some precise Mudras which might be explained.

Chapter 17: Important Information

In this economic ruin, we'll cross over the little tweaks and suggestions that can improve or break the effectiveness of your Mudras. Many people may additionally want to try to perform Mudras with out this understanding, skipping a important element. Let's make certain we in fact recognize how Mudras are correctly finished.

If you definitely choice to attain all of the blessings from Mudras, make certain to take a look at this chapter cautiously from pinnacle to backside so you recognize what to do and what no longer to do.

Timing

The first mistake that people make related to Mudras is that they reduce to rubble the timing of them, in one-of-a-type strategies.

Firstly, pretty some people try to carry out Mudras virtually at night, when they get home after art work or university. Chances are they may be without a doubt exhausted. Therefore this isn't always an splendid idea, as Mudras are appeared to be exceptional used in the path of the early to mid-morning times. It is within the intervening time of the day that people revel in extra calm, relaxed and non violent.

So, ensure to perform a unmarried or more Mudras in the end of the first light in preference to leaving it until the stressful night-time. Don't fear, you don't want to rouse 30 minutes earlier (it's miles as an entire lot as you) because it's enough making an funding 10 minutes, despite the fact that the greater you exercise, the tons less tough and faster you'll get consequences. You really can use them at night time time, in particular the ones Mudras for preventing insomnia (defined later), however have in mind to make investments greater time whilst you wake up.

The special mistake that people make related to timing is concerning the time period they hold each Mudra. Many beginners might imagine that maintaining a Mudra for 1minute is sufficient to gather the blessings that Mudra produces.

Unfortunately, this isn't always real…

According to specialists, it's been proved that 10 to 45 minutes of maintaining Mudras are recommendable so you can paintings at its excellent. There are some exceptions as we will see in some time.

Now, impatience is some element this is found in everybody, however it's miles a few factor that desires to be conquer, the terrific manner to do that is frequently boom the time you spend the usage of Mudras.

If you are a beginner, you can need to begin the use of them for, permit' say, five minutes. Try to be targeted and no longer considering other subjects. If any idea shows up for your mind, genuinely allow it pass, don't try to hold directly to it. Then, bypass decrease once more and popularity in your Mudra.

If you are trying to set off a particular Chakra, you could want to visualize the place of that Chakra on your frame. On the opposite hand, in case you are the usage of a Mudra for weight reduction or any sort of Mudra we can see in a while, focusing in your respiration would be a first rate idea.

FREQUENCY AND POSITION

Another issue that confuses a few humans is the frequency of Mudras. They aren't certain how frequently they need to carry out the Mudra inside the path of the route of the day.

Several human beings have a tendency to think the usage of a Mudra as speedy as an afternoon is sufficient!

While that might be actual if you exercise for 45 or more minutes, that's not the amazing element to do particularly for novices who also can discover slightly difficult to preserve awareness for that time body.

If you perform Mudras, you want to do them in a manner that makes it the most beneficial for you.